PRAISE FOR *THE GUT WELLNESS GUIDE*

"Allison and Stephen have done the miraculous: written a book about the functioning of our bodies in an ever-so-personal and delicious way. They write so clearly and with such warmth and mastery that what seemed obtuse and dry is suddenly understandable, even—dare I say—exciting. And, as a grateful recipient of Allison's hands-on magic, I can say with utter conviction that the love that comes through her work is astounding. It is, after all, love that heals, and now we can all be recipients of that magic through this book."

—GENEEN ROTH, author of the *New York Times* #1 best seller *Women Food and God*

"Through their intimate knowledge of anatomy and extensive hands-on experience, Allison and Stephen gift us with the definitive practical roadmap to a healthy gut, a stronger immune system, increased energy, and a sense of a greater quality of life. Yet the big surprise is that the practice of their simple yet powerful techniques brings us joy."

—GREG HICKS AND RICK FOSTER, best-selling authors of *How We Choose to Be Happy*

"Allison and Stephen have deep knowledge and expertise of both traditional and contemporary healing arts. But more importantly, in this book they point us to our own individual capacity to heal and to rediscover our innate wholeness. Trust your gut, buy this book."

—FRANK OSTASESKI, author of *The Five Invitations: Discovering What Death Can Teach Us About Living Fully*

"Allison and Stephen provide simple, easily applied techniques for accessing the body's self-healing mechanisms and they are very persuasive in their appeal for cultivating a relationship with one's own body in the pursuit of optimal health. Their gentle appeal for a life of greater being is both disarming and at times irresistible."

—ROBERT P. TURNER, MD, holistic psychiatrist

THE

GUT WELLNESS GUIDE

THE POWER OF BREATH, TOUCH, AND AWARENESS
TO REDUCE STRESS, AID DIGESTION, AND RECLAIM
WHOLE-BODY HEALTH

ALLISON POST AND **STEPHEN CAVALIERE**

North Atlantic Books
Berkeley, California

Published by
North Atlantic Books
Berkeley, California

Authors' photo by John L. Hall
Cover design by Rob Johnson
Book design by Happenstance Type-O-Rama

Printed in the United States of America

An earlier version of this book was previously published by North Atlantic Books in 2003 as *Unwinding the Belly: Healing with Gentle Touch*. This edition has been thoroughly revised and updated.

Medical Disclaimer: The following information is intended for general information purposes only. Individuals should always see their health care provider before administering any suggestions made in this book. Any application of the material set forth in the following pages is at the reader's discretion and is his or her sole responsibility.

The Gut Wellness Guide: The Power of Breath, Touch, and Awareness to Reduce Stress, Aid Digestion, and Reclaim Whole-Body Health is sponsored and published by the Society for the Study of Native Arts and Sciences (dba North Atlantic Books), an educational nonprofit based in Berkeley, California, that collaborates with partners to develop cross-cultural perspectives, nurture holistic views of art, science, the humanities, and healing, and seed personal and global transformation by publishing work on the relationship of body, spirit, and nature.

North Atlantic Books' publications are available through most bookstores. For further information, visit our website at www.northatlanticbooks.com or call 800-733-3000.

Library of Congress Cataloging-in-Publication Data

Names: Post, Allison, 1956– author. | Cavaliere, Stephen, 1960– author.
Title: The gut wellness guide : the power of breath, touch, and awareness to reduce stress, aid digestion, and reclaim whole-body health / Allison Post and Stephen Cavaliere ; foreword by Sara Gottfried, MD.
Other titles: Unwinding the belly
Description: Berkeley, California : North Atlantic Books, [2018] | Revision of: Unwinding the belly / Allison Post & Stephen Cavaliere. | Includes bibliographical references and index.
Identifiers: LCCN 2018013884 (print) | LCCN 2018014953 (ebook) | ISBN 9781623172572 (ebook) | ISBN 9781623172565 (paperback)
Subjects: LCSH: Breathing exercises—Therapeutic use. | Stomach—Massage. | Healing. | Self-help techniques. | BISAC: HEALTH & FITNESS / Diseases / Abdominal. | BODY, MIND & SPIRIT / Healing / General. | HEALTH & FITNESS / Healing.
Classification: LCC RM733 (ebook) | LCC RM733 .P67 2018 (print) | DDC 615.8/36—dc23
LC record available at https://lccn.loc.gov/2018013884

1 2 3 4 5 6 7 8 9 KPC 22 21 20 19 18

Printed on recycled paper

North Atlantic Books is committed to the protection of our environment. We partner with FSC-certified printers using soy-based inks and print on recycled paper whenever possible.

*Dip in
to the sea
of possibilities*

—PATTI SMITH

CONTENTS

WITH GRATITUDE | xiii

FOREWORD | xvii

CHAPTER 1: My Path toward Embodiment | 1

Emergencies   2

Emergence   4

Embodiment   7

CHAPTER 2: Your Belly Leading the Way | 9

Intuition   9

Digestion   12

Emotion   17

Movement   21

Other Sources of Tension   23

CHAPTER 3: First Steps in Unwinding—Belly Breathing and Working the Navel, Skin, and Lymph | 27

Belly Breathing   29

Gentle Touch   33

Unwinding the Navel   34

Exploring the Abdominal Surface with the Cat's Paws Touch   36

Lymph Pumping   38

A Note on Anatomy and Physiology   39

CHAPTER 4: Intermediate Steps in Unwinding—
Lateral Breathing and Elimination | **47**

Lateral Breathing   48
Connecting to the Large Intestine (Colon)   53
Bowel Movements and Stools   57

CHAPTER 5: Gut Matters | **67**

A Deeper Understanding   67
The Three Tubes of the Embryo   69
Infection, Immunity, and Imbalance   72
Imbalance, Birth, and Developing Together   74
The Microbiome   76
The Gut Brain   78

CHAPTER 6: Further Steps in Unwinding—
Expanded Lateral Breathing and Digestion | **91**

Expanded Lateral Breathing   91
Stimulating the Digestive Organs   92
Supermarkets and Being Mindful   100

CHAPTER 7: Three-Dimensional Breathing and the Back | **109**

Three-Dimensional Breathing   109
Integrating the Back   110

CHAPTER 8: Advanced Steps in Unwinding—
Connected Breathing, the Inner Voice, and Bone | **123**

Connected Breathing   124
The Inner Voice   128
Intercostals   130
Lower Abdomen   132
Bone   134

CHAPTER 9: An Action Plan for Gut Health | **141**

Toward a Balanced Life   141

A Note on the Action Plan   144

Blood Tests and Metabolic Markers   145

Saying Farewell to Sugar   147

Digging Deeper with a Comprehensive Stool Analysis   149

A Food-Elimination Protocol   151

Making Adjustments While Keeping with Your
        Core Program   154

Deepening Your Embodiment Practice   156

RESOURCES | **161**

INDEX | **165**

ABOUT THE AUTHORS | **179**

ILLUSTRATIONS

CHAPTER 2

2.1 Common sense   11

2.2 Digestion   15

2.3 The viscera   16

2.4 Brain chemistry   18

2.5 Movement   22

2.6 Other sources of tension   24

CHAPTER 3

3.1 Belly breathing   30

3.2 Movement of the diaphragm   32

3.3 The circuit of healing   38

CHAPTER 4

4.1 Lateral Breathing—left side   49

4.2 Lateral Breathing—right side   49

4.3 Full Lateral Breathing   49

4.4 The shape of the relaxed, healthy diaphragm   50

4.5 Enhanced lateral movement   52

4.6 The shape of the relaxed, healthy colon   56

CHAPTER 6

6.1 Digestive organs—left side   95

6.2 Digestive organs—right side   96

CHAPTER 7

7.1 Three-dimensional breathing   110

7.2 Fluid movement   112

7.3 The kidneys and the adrenal glands   113

CHAPTER 8

8.1A Connected breathing   125

8.1B Connected breathing   125

8.2 Intercostals   131

WITH GRATITUDE

Benjamin Sahler, a Jungian psychologist, author, translator, and fellow belly-lover, asked us if we would agree to let him translate into French our first edition of this book, which we called *Unwinding the Belly: Healing with Gentle Touch.* This unsolicited offer from a complete stranger came twelve years after the publication of that book, and so we consider it to have been serendipitous. Benjamin's kind offer was the perfect excuse for a visit to the South of France where we met Benjamin and his wife—and artistic collaborator—Marie Martine. Benjamin's translation and our visit to France inspired us to expand upon the original scope of the work and to create this new offering.

We do so with the encouragement of those who are steeped in the world of the new advances in the science of all things Gut, who now unashamedly point to the vital roles that stress and its mitigation, and the need to pursue a deeper meaning in life, play in the quest for authentic health. That, coupled with the belief that those who are skilled in meditation and spiritual practice now recognize the need to maintain physical health and respect, if not honor, the belly and its ways.

And so it is with gratitude that we extend our love and appreciation to so many good friends and stalwart colleagues who helped us, in one way or another, keep to our truth while fulfilling our pledge to learn more about bellies and more about life.

Specifically, we thank Gilles Marin for being our first and best belly-teacher, Robert Turner for his unfailing moral and professional support, and Sara Gottfried for her generosity of spirit. Rosalie Arcadi, Michael Bellino, Astride Hofmann, Monica Passin, and Susan Skornicka—all friends who were there to listen and offer tangible assistance and encouragement during the challenging decade when we were caregiving for our elderly parents—we feel blessed by their presence.

Over many years Fred Arnicar has proffered just the right touches of dry wit whenever Stephen was in sore need of a fresh perspective, and although Fred will deny it, he is remarkable for being kind. Dan K. Palmer has for several years generously provided a one-room refuge for Stephen to write this and other works. We thank Stewart for sharing his Paris with us, and when Nicole Lambrou clued us in about a certain cozy writer's retreat in San Francisco, we discovered a camaraderie we had yet to experience.

We regard North Atlantic Books as a publishing company that has always been willing to let writers speak their truth and present philosophies not always in the mainstream. We cannot express enough gratitude to them for supporting the effort to get our work out to a larger audience. A special thanks to Sarah Serafimidis for her help with all things French, and for her invitation to us to consider further creative projects with North Atlantic Books. Many thanks to Erin Wiegand for getting the project started in a timely way and to our project leader, Ebonie Ledbetter, for her thoughtful guidance. Thanks also to Hisae Matsuda for her close editorial work and to Diana Salles for her illustrations.

We hope that North Atlantic will continue to fulfill a vital role in the industry, and provide artists who could not otherwise gain visibility with a place to call home.

After having followed up with some of our clients who shared their stories in the first book, we were able to do some updates. (We also added a new story.) But for the most part we have retained the originals because we believe they continue to inspire and reflect the experience of so many others. While these stories may at first strike the reader as too unique and personal, they are remarkable for their breadth of understanding, and so we thought it better to leave them largely unaltered. We are indeed grateful for the honesty and courage of those who have shared their stories with all of us.

Allison wakes up happy each morning, grateful for another day with Stephen. His humor, intelligence, imagination, and enduring commitment to her work and growth continue to amaze her, and she abides in his capacity to listen to, see, and love her.

Stephen has had the pleasure of sharing thirty plus years with Allison, and to this day feels it a gift from on high to partake in her unique and refreshing way of speaking and of being. Over the decades he has also had the pleasure to witness the tenderness and love exchanged between Allison, students, and clients, and it is for this reason that he has chosen to convey the content of this work in her words and in her voice.

We dedicate this book to these very clients and students—and to our readers, whose health and well-being remain our *raison d'être*.

FOREWORD

In 2016, I was referred to Allison Post by one of the leaders in the functional-medicine movement, the type of medicine that I practice. At the time, I had been struggling with mysterious symptoms that conventional medicine hadn't solved. Unfortunately, neither complementary/ alternative medicine nor functional medicine—the form of personalized, predictive, preventive, and participatory medicine that focuses on optimal functioning of the body using a systems-based approach—had improved my symptoms. I landed on Allison's doorstep, perplexed, downtrodden, and not sure where to go next.

Enter the ebullient, energetic being Allison Post. Allison practices a novel form of functional medicine, but I'd take it one step further—she is the next generation of functional medicine, even though she's been in practice for more than thirty years. She is a rare clinician who applies a highly developed medical intuition to listening, gentle visceral touch, and craniosacral therapy. I liken Allison to a wise fairy godmother who happens to be brilliantly versed in Eastern and Western healing arts. Allison has helped thousands of people heal symptoms, from chronic and serious to minor and nagging. And she has certainly helped me.

I had a problem that was all too common: I have a delicate nervous system damaged by too much stress, over-providing, and over-efforting. You too may need a nervous system reset—the way that you know is that your hormones are out of whack, or your gut won't heal, or maybe you can't shake anxiety, depression, or addiction. We all have different vulnerabilities that emerge when the nervous system, or any other system in the body, is overwhelmed. Mine was muscle tension dysphonia. I experienced such tight muscles around my neck, voice box, and diaphragm that I lost my voice. I hit a wall trying to find solutions in a broken, disease-based health-care system. My well-meaning physicians offered me Botox injections into my vocal cords, which hardly seemed like a long-term or palatable option.

What I didn't know before meeting Allison is that I was missing something essential: a set of simple yet time-honored exercises to reconnect with my body, tap into my body's intuitive center, and soothe my overtaxed nervous system. Result? By helping me relearn how to breathe deeply, with more freedom and a softer belly than I've ever learned in my decades of practicing yoga, I've been able to reclaim my health.

Indeed, Allison has more than met my needs for the past year, specific to my constitution and current situation. Further, she has helped me tune into my needs in a way that I was missing before we met. She helps me activate my innate healing response. We do this by understanding what is out of balance, finding the resources to support it, and accessing my ability to grow. And she can do this for you, together with her inspiring husband and partner, Stephen Cavaliere, who not only gives emotional support but works side by side with her, translating her method and supporting the transformation of their clients.

Through health coaching and bodywork, Allison has unfolded different layers of my history and revealed my own ability for healing and change. She's not the type of practitioner you become dependent on; she teaches you so you can become your own healer. When I asked Allison about her work, and how my experience might be similar to other patients or to readers of her book, she replied:

When I first met you, I believed that you had all the Four Ps of Functional Medicine* in place just beautifully, so we went right to slowing down your nervous system and encouraging your inherent health system to realign

---

* Personalized, predictive, preventive, and participatory medicine.

and strengthen. I invite everyone to slow down and gently allow what needs to be met in the moment to bring the nervous system back into balance so we know how to proceed. Often, in a slow and quiet way, I bring people into direct contact with their organs, fluids, and any obstacle, as well as the inherent, healthy flow. Then they can begin to discern their inner landscape.

As part of the masterful revision of *Unwinding the Belly*, Allison and Stephen have added a clear understanding of the new science on the gut, the microbiota and microbiome, and the role that stress, diet, and the physical environment plays—but more important, the effect it has on the nervous system and our relationships to self and to others. You will learn about one of the problems that I've faced and I see so commonly in my own practice, the vicious cycle of gut–nervous, system–stress imbalance.

Just as Allison has helped me, this book will help you. *The Gut Wellness Guide* will teach you how to develop your embodiment skills by breathing, tapping into your internal organs with a gentle touch, and deepening your awareness through feeling. Whether you have chronic pain or your psychiatrist told you to meditate, or you are trying to recover from trauma or injury, or you are searching for gut and digestive relief, or you're like me and need to reset your nervous system, Allison has a proven method here for you. This book is nearly equivalent to seeing her at her office in Marin County, California.

I hope you feel comforted and supported by this book, particularly with Allison and Stephen's wise, warm, inclusive, and often humorous language. As a writer, I'm not sure how they do it, but the narrative style is engaging *and* inspiring, and yet clear *and* accessible. Literally, it will help you melt, to put down the fight, and surrender to the power of true health.

This book belongs in the library of anyone who is frustrated with conventional medicine and is seeking a systems-based form of healing. Functional medicine holds great promise to change mainstream medicine into personalized medicine. I hope that your copy of *The Gut Wellness Guide* becomes one of those rare self-healing books, full of notes and dog-eared pages, that you return to when you need to relieve chronic tension, reset your nervous system, and upgrade your healing.

SARA GOTTFRIED, MD
Berkeley, California

1

My Path toward Embodiment

Whenever I am at a party or other casual social gathering, it is inevitable that someone will approach me and ask: "And what is it that you do?"

Most times I tell the truth: "I'm an integrative medicine health coach."

But sometimes I sense that I'll get that worried look, as if to say, "So does that mean I can't have another piece of chocolate cake?"

So instead I offer a reply that tells a deeper truth. "I talk to people about their bellies. I teach them how to breathe, relax, and be happy."

If the person hasn't run away yet, and wants to find out more, I am then happy to talk more about my passion, although I wait a bit before speaking too specifically about bloating, gas, or other matters of the gut.

I wait to speak of such things because my work does indeed revolve around breathing, relaxing, and being happy. That might strike some as an odd combination, and others as being perfectly obvious. Either way, for many people those things no longer come naturally or easily.

I know this because for more than thirty years I've been helping others navigate stress and the many problems that come with, well, being in a body. Being healthy and feeling authentically good, as an adult, was something I too had lost along the way and had to relearn. Everyone has a different story, and that is as it should be. My work is mostly about listening to others, but my story might have something just enough in common with yours to be of service, so I'll share it here.

EMERGENCIES

I was nineteen in 1975, and I was lying on the beach trying to enjoy the sunshine, the warmth of the sand, and the sound of the waves. But the pain in my belly kept me writhing. It came in sharp thrusts from below my navel. It felt like a wad of tangled rubber bands that were threatening to suddenly pull and snap. Christmas vacation at the beach in Florida turned into a trip to the local hospital.

The doctors had no idea of the cause of my distress, and after issuing painkillers they put me in a room overnight to recover. In the confused atmosphere of the hospital, where it smelled of decay and disinfectant, I had time to think. I had been riddled with infections for the prior two years, since the time I had begun to use the Dalkon Shield. Like many "liberated" young women of the seventies, I had been using the birth control device since my late teens. The standard treatment for the periodic infections was invariably a round of antibiotics: a treatment prescribed with the attitude that infections were normal for a young woman. Lying in the bed at the hospital in Florida, I asked myself some questions: If the antibiotics were supposed to work, but didn't, why take them, and how could a seemingly benign treatment lead to so much pain? And then I realized—I knew positively—that the Dalkon Shield did not belong inside my body. I also realized that the past two years of periodic infections were not normal. This was my first inkling of the fact that modern medicine was not infallible.

The next morning I returned to New York and went to see my doctor as soon as I could. I insisted that he remove the IUD, and he did so. At the time he feared that my current infection could cause complications, so I again underwent heavy dosages of antibiotics. Nevertheless, two weeks later, at my college in upstate New York, I collapsed in pain, and my alarmed roommate took me to the school infirmary, where I remained in a delirium for three days. When my body temperature passed 104 degrees and continued to climb, I was transferred to the local hospital. There the doctors diagnosed pelvic inflammatory disease and said that I was near death. They hooked me up to receive intravenous antibiotics. After one month of this, the doctors told me that I was lucky to be alive. And they told me in vague anatomical terms that I had a tremendous amount of scarring in my pelvis. I was nineteen, it was 1975, and despite my first doubts raised in Florida, I didn't know to ask a lot of questions.

After that emergency, I returned to my daily life, but found no comfort. I had to return to the hospital many times to treat the various complications of the disease. More important, other conditions arose as well: conditions not so acute as to warrant emergency care, but they put me in a chronic state of disquiet. I became bloated after almost every meal and suffered daily from constipation. My energy was flagging. Generally, my digestion was a mess, and my metabolism seemed to be fading away. I consulted my family and friends and complained to anyone who would listen. I didn't get any information that could be of use; no one knew how to help. "Stomach problems" were considered normal, especially for a girl who was a bit on the chubby side. Life was uncomfortable, but everyone seemed to think that if I wasn't laid up in the hospital, it couldn't be all that bad. So, I did what was expected of me—I persevered.

Then a curious thing happened. As my condition continued to worsen, one day something changed. Finally, I was fed up with it all.

I didn't know exactly what I was going to do to get better, but I did promise myself that I was not going to spend the rest of my life in an endless series of doctor's office visits, hospital stays, and emergency room crises. I knew something was wrong with me that was more basic than just the medical consequences of pelvic inflammatory disease, something that went deeper than my symptoms. I realized that my problems stemmed from ignorance and neglect of my body by the doctors and by me. I was motivated to change because even though my problems had started in the reproductive system, it alarmed me that my metabolism, digestive system, energy level, and entire body were adversely affected.

EMERGENCE

First, I tried the entire gamut of dietary regimes. And while I continued to pursue my lifelong interests in music, theatre, and dance, I took up fitness, yoga, and meditation. I also wanted to study anatomy and physiology, but within a holistic context. I wanted to learn how the body worked in a tangible way, and the only way I knew how to do that was to study massage. A few years later, I did in fact become a licensed massage therapist and began to see clients.

Although I helped many people, and found some relief for my own problems, after several years I had to admit I was not making astounding progress. Something was missing, that one last secret, the pot of gold that always seemed to be just over the rainbow.

When working on other people as a massage therapist, I saw that almost everyone I encountered suffered some degree of chronic low energy, weak metabolism, and digestive imbalance. This led me to look beyond all the aches and pains and the nominal reasons why clients were coming for massage. I realized that a person did not have to have my particular set of problems or have a serious health history to be burdened with the curse of fatigue and a "bad stomach."

More important, I looked at what we all had in common in how we lived and how we sought relief. I then realized that all through my emergencies and all along my healing journey, I had been looking for help in substances and programs that lay outside of myself. Within the strict confines of mainstream medicine, I was waiting for doctors to give me the perfect pill or pull off the one last surgical procedure that would finally put all my problems to rest. Within my new career as a complementary therapist, I was grasping for the one secret that would pull off a healing coup and eliminate my (and my client's) conditions. That was the wrong approach. That was the wrong path.

Soon after this discovery, I made two immediate changes. I studied herbal medicine, but I learned to use herbs not in an allopathic, "fix it" manner, but as food integrated into my diet. I learned that herbs (and supplements) are not to be treated casually, but through knowledge and with caution, and I also began to see diet not as temporary regimen for weight loss, but as continuous and long-term medicine.

And then a couple of years later, by good fortune I stumbled onto a Japanese form of touch therapy called Shiatsu, which is based on traditional Chinese acupuncture and the philosophy of Taoism. At that time Shiatsu was nearly unknown, and therefore, thank goodness, the instruction was not overburdened with an allopathic, medical approach to treatment. As in martial arts, it focused on efficiency of movement, self-understanding, and the development of internal energy. Yes, it was about touching people therapeutically, but it was taught largely as a discipline of developing sensitivity to my clients' underlying physical and emotional states.

Shiatsu opened up a whole new way of looking at the natural world and how people related to it, and it inspired me to spend a year at acupuncture school where I was able to learn more about Traditional Chinese Medicine.

Then I began to study a form of abdominal massage called Visceral Manipulation, but from the perspectives of Traditional Chinese Medicine and Taoist insight. This approach encouraged me to tap into the healing power of both my mind and my internal organs. I began to study my own personal, interior universe. I went inside and found that healing would come from the very same source of my pain, my belly.

From the very first day of study my teachers actively encouraged me to teach what I know, in my own way, in my own words. This is one of the hallmarks of the Taoist approach to knowledge: the teaching changes form to best suit the time and place of instruction. Teacher and student (practitioner and client) find themselves in a particular milieu and this must be accounted for.

Many of the ideas contained in this book stem from my intensive study of abdominal massage coupled with meditation. That may sound esoteric but it's important to remember that the approach is always a study in humanity, simplicity, and usefulness. In fact, these methods were so accessible and effective they became the cornerstones of my massage practice. I introduced them to my clients and students, changing the techniques to suit individual needs and abilities.

As I continued on my journey inward, I revisited a form of yoga that was complementary to my bodywork. The emphasis was on the principle of "start where you are," adapting to the situation at hand. I also studied a subtle form of healing called Craniosacral Therapy, which, to put it simply, is a method of going inside, listening meditatively to the very depths of being within the bones, the cerebrospinal fluid, and deeper still. It is here that one perceives the movement of life, and if that movement is inhibited, the practitioner helps it flow again.

Because of this newfound ability to be in flow, I found that when working with others I could direct my full attention to the whole person, and I could open up to really hear the stories that people were telling. It became clear that as life over the years continued to get more stressful for everyone, more and more people were developing digestive and autoimmune problems. People were becoming frustrated with their medical care and so they began to cycle through a series of alternative diets in search of relief, much like I had at the beginning of my transition from emergencies to emergence.

It became clear that in order to really help people, I needed to rekindle my lifelong investigation into what is at the heart of digestive disorders and autoimmune problems. I wanted to search beyond symptoms and find the root causes of illness. I went back to delve deeper into the anatomy and physiology of the gut.

It is for this reason that my clients began to call me "Sherlock," because instead of only doing bodywork and encouraging them to look into improving their nutritional profile and fitness, I started to ask a lot of questions and listen more deeply.

I believe that it is vital to inquire what one has experienced since the beginning, even exploring what has taken place in utero. This provides clues about the particular obstacles that any of us can have as adults. Even when I am meeting with people online during a video chat, I am able to guide a person to uncover what might be causing their particular conditions, while at the same time working with them to ease tension and unwind any trauma. I show people how to relax and unwind through their breath, guide their touch to make contact with their torsos and bellies, and build upon whatever experience they may have in meditation. Sometimes I introduce more pointed embodiment explorations that answer their individual tension.

Whenever I have an overflow of interest, Stephen and I team up to teach small groups. Curiously, there seems to be no shortage of people desiring to feel better, or at least wondering how the belly fits into that.

When my clients begin to find answers and they need help with things that are beyond my area of expertise, I point them in the direction of where they might be able to find more specific help. Throughout the years I have assembled a posse of practitioners to refer to: functional and integrative medicine doctors, osteopaths, acupuncturists, homeopaths, psychiatrists, and counselors.

And so it is in this way I have evolved from a young woman who had only wanted to dance and sing into someone who is dedicated to helping others overcome obstacles.

EMBODIMENT

Yet even with help, things take time. You cannot get to the root causes, overcome obstacles, and move into flow so quickly, so easily, so deeply.

First it is necessary to unwind and settle inside of yourself. We unravel the confused patterns of movement and the sources of tension that create them: physical, mental, and emotional. After you get more and more comfortable being in your body, feeling it from the inside without mental chatter, and listen to it, you open up to learning more about the biology of your gut and the important ways it affects your health. And then once again you sink into a deeper level of embodiment and health. As your journey unfolds, it will be in a way that is aligned to your health and to your life.

I call my way to embody, to access these deeper levels, "Unwinding." For me it is a practice of going deep and settling into my body, with breath, touch, and awareness. At the same time, I continue being aware of the space around me that supports a larger field of experience so I don't get caught up and tangled in the internal space. I combine that practice with a continuous tweaking of my diet based on how I am feeling, along with study of the biology of the gut. Yet I must emphasize that, lest you get too caught up with chasing answers outside of yourself, the breathing, the sensing, and the feeling is crucial. A gentle embodiment practice, which I call Unwinding, but which you can call anything you like, needs to be cultivated and practiced at least a little bit each day.

As soon as I started on this internal path, my life changed dramatically. During my journey inward to my center, with my center, to better health and self-empowerment, I was able to figure out what activities and pursuits truly work for me. I became healthier and happier than I had ever been. This work has been so incredibly powerful for me as a practitioner that I now teach others how to do it on themselves, and I developed Unwinding to truly help other people to learn, to feel, and to heal, *and* to find joy in the process.

After a healing journey of more than forty years, I offer this book to you. I want to show you things that you can use for yourself. I don't want to linger on abstraction, but give you a map to guide you to the fundamentals, to what is at the core of self-healing. I hope that you can use these ideas and techniques to walk the path of healing and happiness, with the self-respect and the joy that is your birthright, your belly leading the way.

2

Your Belly Leading the Way

It sounds odd, doesn't it? *Your belly leading the way.* But I couldn't be more serious. When anything occurs that is going to affect my body and the way I feel, whether it is an activity, work, communicating with others, or making a decision, I check in with my belly. I let it lead the way.

INTUITION

I want physical health in the present moment. In fact, that's one and the same thing: to be healthy is to be present. I won't settle for an abstract, intangible ideal of health, nor will I be lured by promises of a future state of perfection. I want a way to be comfortable and vital here and now, and the most effective way I know to make it happen, to make health real for me, is to go deep within. If I am willing to feel and listen to my body, I can never be led too far astray. Health is acknowledging, feeling, trusting, and nurturing the intuitive sense that resides in the center.

This intuitive sense is not illusive, nor is it intangible. It is more than a mere concept or a belief, or something to just read about in books. Intuition is exactly what we say when talking honestly to one another: "gut instincts." And like the guts themselves, intuition is entirely tangible. We can touch it, feel it, and use it, because it's right there in our belly.

So what do I mean by being "real" and "in the present"? Well, it's about coming down, coming back inside. We all love to go out there in la-la land, the imaginary world of ideas and thoughts and fantasies and other people's "facts." Yes, it's very enticing and often fun to travel outside, in a disembodied state, to see what's out there. But go too far, as is inevitable, and you get lost. Spend too much time out of your body and it starts to bump into things, becomes flighty or sluggish, and gets confused. And then it starts to complain in the form of weakness or pain. Spend too much time out of your body and it's awfully difficult to remember who you really are in the present moment. Health takes place in the here and now of the physical universe of your body. Without health, it's pretty difficult to find the stability and comfort required for the journey to discover who you are in the larger, more spiritual sense.

Unfortunately, intuition has had a bad reputation in the past few centuries. We have been taught to mistrust ourselves because we have been told that facts derived from medical research are more trustworthy, truer in some way than our intuition. But it isn't fair to compare "cold, hard facts" against intuition. What medical, psychological, or even social studies often demonstrate is the fallibility of human perception that is informed not by intuition, but by "common sense." Yes indeed, common sense is often faulty. It is all the things we say we know because we heard them to be so from everybody around us. Common sense is only a matter of repeating things we've heard and not really thinking about them logically and going inside and listening. That is, we have opinions that are unexamined, but we take comfort in the fact that they are common.

Before deciding what the facts are, we need to listen for a resonance between what we are hearing around us and what we know to be true within us. To be influenced by others is natural, even inevitable, I suppose, and is not always unhelpful, but it must harmonize with our intuition. (Many times intuition is telling us we don't have enough information to know what's what or to make a decision.)

I do believe the scientific quest for truth is a wonderful tool to keep us on track with reality, but science was never meant to suppress our personal

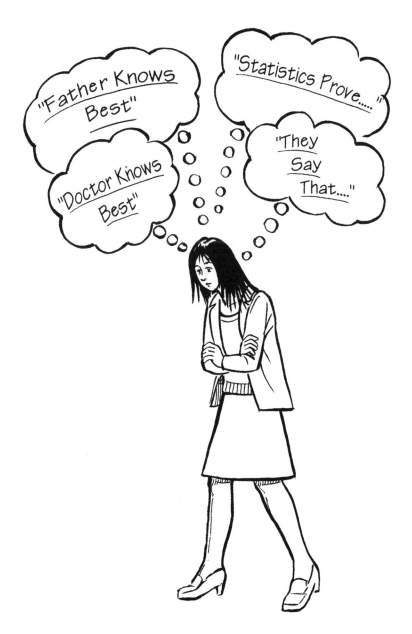

2.1. Common sense. Common sense is based on the opinions of others, which are sometimes used to mislead, and most times created willy-nilly. Dependence upon common sense leads to faulty perception of reality. Inside, you know better.

power. When medical "facts" and dubious studies are trotted out to convince you that you shouldn't trust yourself, well ... that's unfortunate. Opinions from others, even when disguised as science, cannot determine what you experience in the present moment. Intuition comes from within. You, and only you, can be in your center. You just have to be willing to go inside, inhabit your body, and be present. Hey, if you are not in there, who is?

I am, for better or for worse, the living organism that I grew to be. My body is the expression of who I've been and who I am right now. If I can just feel my body instead of wishing it were something different, then I can accept it. If I can move with it instead of forcing it to do things it really doesn't want to do, denying its demands, ignoring the laws by which it functions, then my body ceases to be my enemy. It becomes a source of wonder. It's like a dance where both partners like the music and know the steps. But in this dance my body is an active and knowledgeable partner. It is attuned to the music of internal biorhythms, the seasons, and the timely unfolding of the natural world. Once the trust is there and the dance is going along well, the body naturally seeks what is beneficial to itself, that is, to you. So, to be a good dance partner, it's necessary for you to be present, to listen, to stay in step, and to be guided.

This book is about how to tap the power of your intuition by nurturing the vitality of the physical belly, to use your guts in positive ways for health and happiness.

All well and good, but two questions arise: Why, specifically, is the center so vital to health, and why is it that we often don't trust the belly to lead the way?

Briefly, the center of our body is the focal point of our digestion, our emotional life, and our expressive movement, and these aspects of life can be challenging, to say the least. Let me explain.

DIGESTION

Think about it. What is happening when you feel low on energy? You need food, and so you eat. Where does the food go after you've swallowed it? First, into your stomach, which is tucked up underneath the ribs on the left side. This is where food undergoes its first, substantial breakdown, which can take from twenty minutes to eight hours, depending on the type of food you have eaten and how you have combined it.

Then the food is off to the small intestine, the narrow tube that winds and curls back and forth, covering the area of the midsection, behind the navel. Put your hand on your belly, covering the navel with the palm spread. That is the general area, although a little wider and deeper, where the roughly twenty feet of the thin tube of the small intestine lives. It is here in the center that food is absorbed into the blood to be transported to the other organs of the belly and then miraculously transformed into ... you!

Almost everything you eat becomes, for better or worse, the organs, bone, blood, muscle, skin, and all the other tissues of your body. Every cell of your body is nourished by the energy garnered from the food absorbed by the small intestine. Your body cannot function well or even survive for very long without a steady supply of food energy.

The belly is home to other vital organs that keep you alive and constitute much of what you are internally, in the physical sense. Collectively, these organs are known as the viscera. So when I say "the belly" I'm not only talking about the small intestine, but also the liver, gallbladder, spleen, pancreas, stomach, large intestine (colon), kidneys, ureters, and bladder. These are the organs of digestion and elimination. Usually we don't give these parts of our body the slightest thought. Given the fact that they constitute a very large part of what we are, they certainly deserve more attention.

Within the belly there are many other important, secondary structures not directly connected with the digestion. These include the reproductive organs, the peritoneum and mesentery (tissue that hold things in place) and the various muscles and layers of skin that make up the outer trunk. There is also the blood within its vessels, transporting nutrients, various bundles of nerve tissue connecting to the spine, and layers of lymph that carry away much of the body waste.

Have I forgotten anything? I probably did. Anatomically the center is very complex and it is useful to study it in detail. But it is not essential at this point. To be healthy you want to recognize and respect the belly's vital role in the digestion of food energy and elimination of waste. Ignore this at your peril. Use it to your benefit.

All the various tissues of the body—the blood, bones, muscles, skin, cartilage, fascia, eyes, hair, (and let's not forget the brain!)—rely on the viscera to transform food energy into every element you need to keep you alive and well. The internal organs either use the energy, share surpluses with other organs that may be deficient, or store excesses if there is an overload. The viscera build, repair, and defend the body while maintaining their own integrity. But they can do all this in an effective way only if they are healthy, robust, and unobstructed.

Toxicity from tension, stagnant build-up of waste products, inherent tissue weakness, and stress can congest the center. If the small intestine is overloaded the entire body can become fatigued, tight, uncomfortable, even painful. To feel our best, the small intestine has to be able to do its job. Food should nourish the body instead of adding to a backlog of burdening waste product. If we wish to replenish ourselves with food, we should be ready to receive it with a clear center.

But unfortunately, most often it is not clear. One reason we do not trust what our body is telling us (listen to our intuition) is that we don't like what it has to say! There is a lot of painful stress down there and we avoid acknowledging it. We fill our bellies with an incredible variety (and sometimes quantity) of food, in complicated combinations, and demand that our body assimilate with no complaint. We eat whatever we want, whenever we want, however we want. And we never touch our belly or help it out in any way.

The small intestine contorts and twists, trying to adjust, to adapt, and to do its job the best it can. Then it clogs up with toxicity, hurts even more, and now we really don't want to feel it! We continue with our habits and then wonder why our body seems to be slowly and steadily breaking down.

Because we have learned to ignore the belly, it is no great mystery how we become confused about what constitutes a proper diet. When we try to change our eating habits for the better, we begin to make contact with the

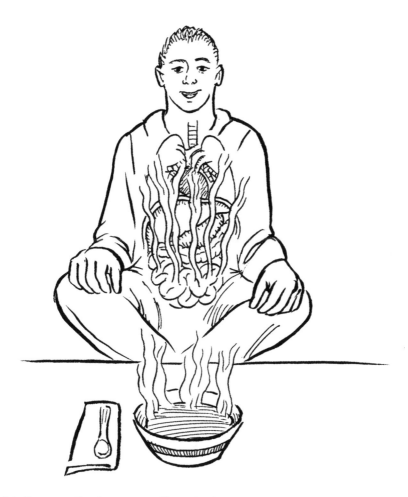

2.2. Digestion. Food energy is efficiently absorbed in, and transported from, a relaxed belly.

center. At the beginning, and possibly for some time, it doesn't feel good. This understandably leads to frustration and a feeling of hopelessness about our diet. It becomes hard to distinguish between good and harmful food. Trapped in this kind of scenario, it's very tempting to blame everything on the aging process. But deep down we don't believe it. Our belly is saying "ouch" and we know it's for a good reason.

To clear the channels of communication, to get in touch with the intuitive center, you need to soften, detoxify, and unwind the tissues in the belly. If you want health, you have to initiate a receptive relationship with your small intestine and the other organs of the digestive and eliminative center; that is, you have to feel your viscera. It may not sound very glamorous, but it's very effective, and it's the least you can do, considering all the work your guts do for you.

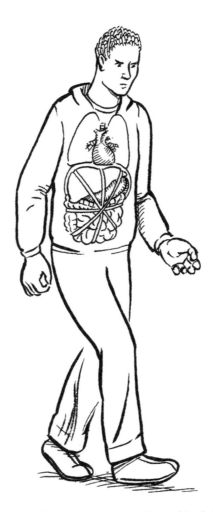

2.3. *The viscera.* Abuse, neglect, contraction, and pain block digestion and access to intuition.

EMOTION

I know that the current popular thinking is that the emotions are governed by brain chemistry. But this leaves something out, doesn't it? What governs brain chemistry? Say what you will, but all those chemicals sloshing about your brain came from food energy, from the center. The brain's chemistry certainly does affect the body, but its functioning also reflects the state of the body. Energy from food, physical activity, the learning environment, and emotional states all arise within the body and affect the brain, but food energy does so most immediately.

For example, imagine spending a week on a desert island with no readily available source of food or water. In this scenario you will experience some interesting changes in brain chemistry, and those, in turn, will affect your thoughts, feelings, and will to move. But it's the lack of food and water that is the most basic.

As novel and fascinating as they are, to know the physiological details of brain mechanism won't really help you on a desert island. Relying on artificial, synthetic interventions in the form of pills in an attempt to govern brain function won't help either. Of course there are cases that require a temporary intervention, but long-term reliance is not really healing, is it? And so it is in our normal, daily life. Knowing all about the brain and using medication cannot help, in the long haul, to improve fitness or live a full, emotionally rich life.

The center does more than assimilate food energy; it is also home to the emotions—digesting them, eliminating some, and enjoying others. If you want to feel, and want to feel good, go to your belly.

We already know that the emotions arise in the body. It is in our common language. It is proverbial that emotions manifest in the center. I've talked about gut intuition, and we know we also have gut feelings. When we feel something very strongly we say we feel it viscerally. We have butterflies in our stomachs and our hearts break. When we experience unexpected and intense fear we feel the need to urinate or evacuate—even before we are aware of the cause of our fear. Worry can eat away at our stomachs, jealousy can waste away the liver, and we lose control and vent our spleen. These are just a few examples of what is obvious to people who still speak the colloquial tongue. We don't normally think of the emotions as bodily functions, but that's the way we experience them, and that's the way we feel them.

Of course, this may not be obvious to some of us. We have the habit of speaking about our physiology in scientific jargon, and that jargon, for its own valid reasons, excludes discussion of the emotions. Traditionally, study of the emotional life has been relegated to a branch of the study of the mind. Here too the mind, like the brain, is too often seen as a disembodied, independent entity with the job of governing the emotions.

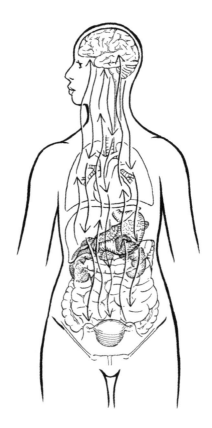

2.4. Brain chemistry. Brain chemistry reflects the state of the rest of the body and its optimal function is part and parcel of bodily health.

What's so tricky about emotions is that they can't be observed with a microscope. They are hard to define and think about. They change and flit about like the wind. But that is certainly no reason to exclude them from the quest for health, or to believe that we can control them merely by manipulating their shadows—brain chemistry. Regardless of all that can be argued about this, we know deep down that the emotions are experienced in the body, especially within the viscera. More important, when they are felt rather than merely talked about, they can be worked with.

We experience some emotions, such as grief and love in the higher organs, particularly the lungs and heart. When this happens, they are difficult to deny for very long without consequences. The emotional charge of unresolved or unexpressed grief and love is stored in the tissue surrounding these organs and cannot be stored without evident pain. If the emotion continues to be held inside, without expression, the muscle and fascia become stiff and blocked, inhibiting the physiological functions of these organs. For example, we know that unrequited love can break a heart. When a person will not allow it to break (allowing the energy to drain off), physical symptoms of stress arise, such as hardening of the arteries and high blood pressure. Of course, there are no hard and fast rules that connect particular organ systems with the expression of specific emotions. How distress manifests depends on individual proclivities. But it is certain that disturbed emotion will affect the body and mind in some way.

Other emotions arise in the viscera, and they too can become stuck. Unfelt, unacknowledged, or otherwise not-honored sensations and feelings are stored in the interconnecting fascia (mesentery), the lining surrounding the viscera (peritoneum), the surrounding layers of skin and muscle, and within the organs themselves. Anger, fear, sadness, and worry can get buried and forgotten in the tissues. It takes effort (and energy) to contain these emotions and that inevitably drains a person. Tightness, fatigue, pain, and, eventually, the various symptoms of physical disease will manifest. Too much undigested emotion, over the long run, can make us sick just in the same way as too much undigested food can.

I don't want you to think that I'm concerned here with only negative emotions. Please don't think that if you touch your belly you will go around endlessly weeping in the streets. Spontaneous desires, joy, a bubbling sense of delight in our own existence, and other positive emotions arise in the belly as well. They come welling up from our center into our consciousness. Isn't it always a pleasant surprise when that happens? Don't we often say: "I'm feeling great, just because ..."? However, we often also block the expression of positive emotions (sometimes by tightening our abdomens.) Have you ever found yourself in a situation where you had to restrain a sudden sense of pure joy, compassionate love, excitement, or desire? That's just about every day for most people. But no matter how many good marks you receive for your restrained behavior, over the long run, always being polite turns into the ingrained habits of a lackluster life, and worse, into deep-seated frustration. The hallmark of frustration is contraction and tightness, especially in the neck. But I bet you can guess where I think the root of all that tension is held!

When people try to change the way they feel, to combat frustration or depression, for example, they usually first try to change their thoughts. They attempt to use their minds like a computer, changing thought-input to produce different feeling-output. But these valiant efforts are in vain. It's necessary, first, to check into the center to find out exactly which raw feelings are really stuck there, where they are stuck, and if they are in reaction to present conditions or to old, outdated, stale memories. Then you must do the things that will physically clear the way for the free flow of information to the rest of the body and to your psyche.

We all would like to reason out our problems without feeling bad. The thinking mind will try to disconnect from the center and attempt to do the job of feeling better on its own. Or it will try to censor the emotional content coming from the belly. Unfortunately, we can't pick and choose to feel only the good or safe emotions and banish the rest. It's an all-or-nothing system. If you want the really authentic goodies, you'll have to honor the not so good feelings that are a part of life. You have to feel them, not think them, even though many people confuse thinking about emotions with feeling them. I guess everyone goes through that stage in life where they believe that if they could just figure everything out, all would be well. But there's no protection in a purely mental world. That's not the way the body likes to do things. It wants to feel. Here's a secret: when emotion is truly felt, without layers of interpretation, it quickly dissipates. For it truly is like the wind.

So the center is the physical nexus of the emotions, the good, the bad, and the indifferent. It is the place where we feel our way through life. Unwinding your belly will restore the holistic conversation between the feeling body and thinking mind. It clears the center of obstructions and allows the free flow of authentic emotion. Only then can we experience life in a complete way: through our feeling, to our healing, the belly leading the way.

MOVEMENT

When our belly leads the way, we follow. When we follow, we move. The belly is the place where we gather and transform food and contact our emotions. Then we take the energy from those two sources and translate it into movement. The center is the springboard for physical movement, the expression of our being in time and space.

Generally, we think of movement propelled by the action of our muscles and bones. That is what we see, on the gross, physical level, when we watch someone else move. We see their limbs making big motions to get the body from point to point, so it's natural to think of the muscles, the bones, and the joints as the origin. We mistake the visible means of movement for the force behind it. But the muscle contractions that move the trunk and limbs (and sometimes even the head) are a reaction to the movement of—let's call it the inner spirit, or inner gumption, if you prefer—and it emanates from a delightful source within the belly.

The next time you have the opportunity to watch your favorite athlete, focus on her belly. At first it isn't obvious that she is moving from her center because we're impressed with the sight of well-toned muscles and distracted by the movements of her limbs. So it's natural to conclude that muscles alone are responsible for her amazing results. However, if you observe the performance by watching her belly closely, you will see that her legs are only an extension of her belly, moving it around where it wants to go. You will see that her trunk and her arms too are moving around the pivot point of her center, doing its bidding. This may be easier to perceive if you first watch a professional dancer, and then again watch your favorite athlete in action. You will see that the motion of the body begins in the center and that the true power of movement can come with much less effort.

This is the main reason, beyond lack of fitness and inadequate warm-up, that weekend warriors, when playing sports, become so sore and frequently injure themselves. They haven't learned how to move freely from their center. To test this concept, try repeatedly hitting a ball against a wall with a tennis

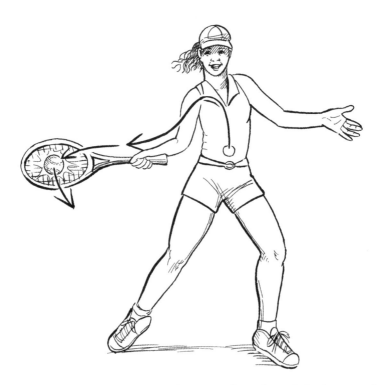

2.5. Movement. Movement starts in the center, flows through the joints, and creates visible action.

racket. Keep swinging the racket while restraining your hips from moving. To accentuate this stiff feeling, try to hit the ball as hard as you can while keeping a stiff belly by holding in your abdominal muscles. I don't recommend you continue this for very long because your arm, shoulder, and back muscles will become exhausted and your joints will begin to hurt. If this way of hitting a tennis ball or other sports motion has become habitual in your game, I can guarantee that you will develop tendinitis, if not other injuries. Regrettably, you will eventually have to give up the sport dear to your heart. At this point you have a choice: you can either blame it on age or you can learn to move from your center.

This isn't only true for tennis or other sports, but for any activity. I relearned this concept in massage school. I say relearned because every healthy infant knows how to move ergonomically; it doesn't have beefy muscles to depend on. The idea of moving from the center came as such a revelation to me that I began to do everything that way, even washing the dishes! So you don't have to be a sports star to tap into the movement power of the belly. You can practice this even when doing the housework. For example, you are not forever condemned to jerk the vacuum cleaner around, or rather, suffer it tossing you around. If you move from your center you will literally be dancing with it. Let the center of your body lead the vacuum to where you want it to go, and once you get the hang of it—no more sore arms! With this kind of movement, even housework can be pleasurable. Well, almost.

OTHER SOURCES OF TENSION

Besides the fundamental tensions related to problems digesting food, feeling emotion, and moving from the center, there are many other, secondary ways the belly can become wound up with tension. Some are common to us all, and some are unique to each individual, so you will have to judge which ones apply specifically to you. As you practice the various techniques of Unwinding that are described in this book, you will be learning invaluable skills to cope with these problems.

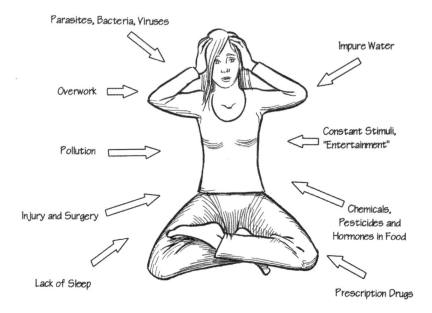

Parasites, Bacteria, Viruses

Impure Water

Overwork

Constant Stimuli, "Entertainment"

Pollution

Injury and Surgery

Chemicals, Pesticides and Hormones in Food

Lack of Sleep

Prescription Drugs

2.6. Other sources of tension.

Toxicity can collect in the body from outside sources of pollution: from impure air, water, and the vast number of toxic chemicals, antibiotics, and artificial hormones used to grow and preserve food. All medications and over-the-counter drugs have residual side effects that collect in the various tissues of the viscera, especially the liver. The shock of surgery can affect the body, chemically and emotionally. Surgical scar tissue can block the free flow of blood, nutrients, and nerve conduction. Lack of proper exercise, without question, is a major source of toxicity, and extra body weight from inactivity burdens the entire system. Lack of deep sleep and overwork are also two common, and increasing, sources of tension. Added to that is the tension created by constant, unrelenting exposure to outside stimuli. It is very difficult for the body to process what is on the inside while it is reacting to the bombardment of sounds, images, and sensations that we currently take for granted as the normal way of life. Finally, the body is continually defending itself against harmful bacteria, viruses, and parasites from the environment.

When you think about it, it's amazing how much the body deals with on a daily basis! And I'm sure I've left out several things. Wouldn't it be nice to help out your body a little by reducing the tension that you carry around?

These are all well-known sources of stress. You can fill libraries with the books written on the specific (sometimes too specific) therapies devised to combat them. But I want to offer you the idea that the simple system of Unwinding is designed to complement any therapy you may be engaged in right now. In fact, even though this may be controversial, I believe that such therapies can actually be ineffective, even detrimental, without first (or concurrently) clearing and bringing tonicity to the center with inner awareness and touch. That's what I found to be true in my personal healing journey and why I'm writing this book.

You may think it odd that I consider all these problems secondary. The current thinking is that these stressors are the fundamental source of all the problems that most people in our society face today. But I feel that to help resolve these problems it's vital to first step behind them, to get underneath them, so to speak, to first connect with your individual source of tension and the center of vitality, the belly. That's where the root of health is.

There are things that you can do about most problems, even if you don't yet know what they are, but it's wise to start with smaller things at the beginning of your healing journey before getting swept up in problems beyond your control. I encourage you to start with, or certainly not neglect, the personal healing that comes with Unwinding, and make that your point of departure.

3

First Steps in Unwinding– Belly Breathing and Working the Navel, Skin, and Lymph

Whenever one of my clients is having a difficult time with digestion, movement, connecting with her body or her true emotion, or when she finds herself in a rut, struggling with healing, I notice that she has in some way constricted her breathing. Rather than get entangled in the web of her apparent problems, I gently repeat one of my personal mantras: "Breathing is so groovy," and I go to the belly, because that is where true breathing begins.

People often ask me: Why is breathing so important? Doesn't everyone breathe? Isn't it just something we do naturally? Here are my short answers to these questions.

Belly-breathing is important, even vital, because it puts you immediately back into your body and helps you feel fully, from the center outward to the extremities. If you are breathing into your belly, which is the natural way, it's almost impossible to remain stressed and uncomfortable.

Yes, everyone does breathe, but very few people do so anywhere near full potential. Almost everyone I encounter is breathing just enough to stay alive and no more.

Though we all may have started out with full, healthy breathing (witness how a healthy newborn child's abdomen moves up and down) we eventually learned from those around us how to be stressed, panicked, upset, disconnected, and in too much of a hurry to take the time for full, even breaths. At best, we fill only the top portion of our lungs, panting our way through life.

We didn't start out like this. We had to learn how to act this way. But we don't have to continue to do anything that makes us uncomfortable and unhappy. Suffocating on stale air is a bad drug if there ever was one. To breathe in a short, limited, gasping, and self-inhibiting fashion may be common, but it is not the way it has to be for you.

When you relearn how to breathe deeply, fully, with freedom, you will reap amazing benefits. It's just a matter of giving yourself this gift. Don't you deserve a full, continuous, clear supply of fresh air? Did you do something wrong or somehow forfeit your fair share of life-giving oxygen? You deserve to breathe to your full capacity because you are alive and part of this world, and quite frankly, there is truly no way to be healthy and happy without breathing freely.

Many believe they breathe just fine, and are taken aback by the concept of relearning how to breathe. But I don't want to linger on why we must reacquaint ourselves with something that is so natural. It is better to demonstrate what proper breathing actually is. No matter how thorough, exact, or even poetic my arguments on breathing may be, none of them can make you healthy. Doing the right things and experiencing them by feeling while you're doing is what will bring about positive change. If you feel disconnected from your body, out of sorts, unhealthy, or uncomfortable, I can guarantee that, along with whatever other symptoms you have, you are not breathing to your God-given, natural capacity. So let's begin with the first practical step of Unwinding. And whenever you are stressed out, remember my mantra: Breathing is so groovy!

Breathing is a vast and fascinating subject, so we are going to work with it in stages. This will involve actually trying out new ways of breathing, following my instructions. Many of you already know much about breathing, and I congratulate you on your previous study, but I encourage you not to skip this initial step. If you are already practicing a system of self-healing, you already know that it's beneficial to start each practice session with a breathing exercise of some sort. So there is no risk in trying it my way for now. If you don't like it, you can always take up your way again. For those of you who have no idea what breathing is all about, here is a basic, no-stress, simple way to begin.

BELLY BREATHING

Lie on your back with your knees up, either on the bed or the floor. Make sure you are comfortable and that you are in a well-ventilated area. If you wish, you can put pillows under your knees, but make sure you use enough to get your knees well elevated. An alternative is to let your knees come together and rest against each other. You want to be able to relax the legs while not exerting the slightest muscular tension in the hips or abdomen to keep them up.

First, bring awareness to the way you are breathing now. Does it flow, struggle, get caught in your throat or chest? Or is it imperceptible? Is it deep or shallow? Is it painful or boring to rest, to be quiet, to feel your inner rhythm?

Feel your back against the floor. Bring your awareness to your spine. Feel its full length, from the sacrum up through the neck. Keep breathing and connecting to the sensation of your spine.

Place your hands firmly but gently on your belly, index fingers pointing in toward each other, touching the navel, and if you can, keep your elbows resting on the floor.

Inhale slowly, and feel your belly rise gently, pushing against your hands. Exhale and let the belly fall back. Once you have that rhythm in place, with the belly enlarging on the inhale and collapsing on the exhale, try to expand the volume of air taken on the inhale. On each inhale try to fill up the entire belly from your hips up to the bottom edge of the rib cage. Let your chest relax. Try to get the belly to fill up completely, rising on the inhale, lowering on the exhale, without using the chest muscles (fig. 3.1).

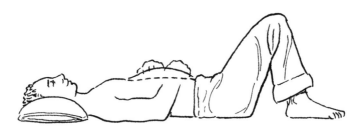

3.1. Belly breathing. Belly Breathing is a soft, pleasant rising and falling of the abdomen. The shoulders, back, neck, upper chest, and surface abdominal muscles stay relaxed.

The more you practice, the more you will grasp this gentle, natural way of breathing. Your belly fills and empties of air almost of its own free will. You want to be careful that you are actually drawing air in deeply to the center, not just flexing the abdominal muscles and pushing the surface out. That's not bringing in air; that's just an abdominal exercise, and it will only make you more tense. Let the air wash in and out as if it were the waves at the seashore. The waves come in and out of their own accord—no pumping, no forcing—and in the same way, experience your belly expanding and collapsing as a reaction to the movement of the waves of air.

Another important aspect of Belly Breathing is to breathe in through the nose, and gently—without forcing—to exhale through the mouth. You will have to inhale slowly and gently, and relax all muscles, in order to fill up the belly entirely. Exhale through the open mouth in an unhurried fashion and soften the neck and jaw. (You don't want to be exhaling through clenched teeth.) Quite often people hear "open the mouth," and instead of letting go of tension in the jaw, they purse the lips and blow hard. That's not it. Let the jaw drop, and on the exhale, give a gentle sigh.

All this may take some practice. Don't expect to get it all at once. Check to see where it is difficult to fill up with breath and if you can do it without muscle exertion. (Of course, there are some muscles working, but in very subtle ways.) The softer you keep your legs, back, shoulders, neck, and even the arms, the more air you are going to get in and the more space you will give the internal organs to unwind and expand into. The more relaxed and complete the exhale, the more you will clear the body of old stale air.

When you feel that your breathing is rhythmic, complete, and effortless, you can, at the very end of the exhale, tuck in the abdominal muscles very slightly to expel that last bit of stale air. But be sure to relax the muscles on the subsequent inhale.

If you become dizzy or nauseous, take a rest. Do not be alarmed. It just shows how much you need to do this! Enhanced breathing brings waste products into the bloodstream quite rapidly, and that can make you feel queasy for a bit. If you stay relaxed during this exercise and take it slowly, you will detoxify the blood at a proper pace without any harm whatsoever. If you do become lightheaded, rest until you feel grounded. You can resume your practice at another time.

Despite how simple this exercise may seem or how involved my description is, I urge you not to skip it. Keep practicing until you get the hang of it. When you are comfortable with Belly Breathing you will be energized and will look forward to more. If you find yourself skipping this or the other breathing exercises, I believe you are not going to benefit from the touch techniques or get much value from the other information in this book.

Also, please remember that Belly Breathing is an exercise. It is designed to clear the center of toxicity and to teach the body to breathe naturally. Belly Breathing is not meant to be an ideal form of "perfect" breathing that you are required to do continuously.

Understanding Belly Breathing

Belly Breathing may be awkward at first and can be difficult to learn. That's because we learn most kinesthetic actions by unconscious imitation. The natural, but uncommon, mechanics of breathing are not entirely visible to the naked eye, so proper breathing has to be felt internally, in a specific physical sense. The main muscle of breathing, the diaphragm, works differently than the other muscles of the body. Generally, it makes a horizontal surface within the rib cage, separating your heart and lungs from your viscera, and during a proper inhale it moves down, increasing the pressure in the abdomen and massaging the viscera. This is what makes the belly protrude on the inhale. The increase in pressure below the diaphragm creates a vacuum in the lung cavities (above the diaphragm) and as we all know, nature abhors a vacuum. Air rushes in from the outside to fill this void. When the diaphragm moves down, the deep lobes of the lung (the parts with the most surface area) are supplied with ample oxygen (fig. 3.2).

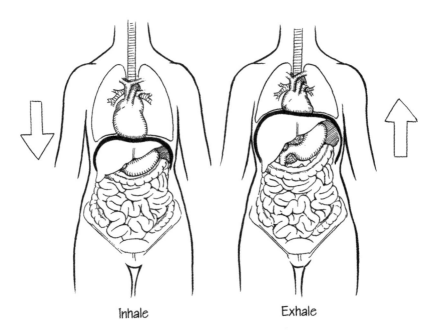

Inhale   Exhale

3.2. *Movement of the diaphragm.* The diaphragm moves down when inhaling, and relaxes up when exhaling.

Unnatural, or what I call panic breath, occurs when the diaphragm is pulled upward on the inhale, and there is much less of a vacuum created, or none at all. This kind of breathing fills only the top lobes of the lungs with oxygen. The body attempts to make up for this lack by contracting the chest and ribcage muscles to expand the lungs. This is the root of neck, shoulder, and back pain. Worse, inadequate breathing deprives the organs and the entire body of its mainstay—vital oxygen. Later, we will discuss why chest breathing is a difficult habit to break and why it may feel uncomfortable to breathe into the belly, even though it is so beneficial.

During this exercise you may have felt spasms and various tight places in the body. Don't worry, that's good! Breathing did not cause this; it only made you capable of feeling the tension that is already there. The first step in restoring your health is increased awareness. Now you know if your body is fatigued and where it is tight. You also know whether it is in need of rest, a good stretch, or exercise. You no longer need anyone else to tell you what you are feeling, what is "wrong" with you, or to nag you to change. Breath brings awareness, and awareness brings action.

Since proper breathing is perhaps the most vital aspect of basic health, we will continue to practice it throughout this book, expanding the reach of relaxed, unforced breathing. After years of neglect and being taken for granted your body is going to really appreciate this new lease on life. But because of the neglect, this new way of enhanced breathing can be very difficult, and the emotional charge can be somewhat threatening. So, like every worthwhile activity in life, it is best to adapt to it slowly. I must repeat that it is best to approach this gently, unhurried, without forcing it. Practice this first step until you are comfortable with it, and then continue on your way to restoring your health.

GENTLE TOUCH

Before moving on to the first touch techniques, I want to remind you to go about all the steps that are presented in this book with an open, curious attitude and a loving presence of mind. Imagine that your hands are the hands of a warm, nurturing, grandmotherly type of woman. If that image doesn't work for you, make up another.

As with the breathing, we will unwind in gentle stages. I feel that the body on a healing journey feels like the unfolding of a living plant. As you know, plants don't just suddenly pop out onto the scene. They take their time—the time best suited to their individual character and circumstances, with each phase of growth developing at its own pace. That's why you will want to proceed with a series of natural stages of organic growth, regardless of how simple it seems or no matter how impatient you may be. I know how it is to want to get out of pain and the rut of ill health as quickly as possible. But the art of healing is the art of taking the time to listen to your body as if it were a rare and precious plant, waiting to flower. Healing is also the art of slowing down. Let's begin.

UNWINDING THE NAVEL

Use the same position as for Belly Breathing. Make sure that you are not holding up your legs with muscle exertion. If you are straining your legs, the hips cannot relax.

With two fingers of whichever hand is comfortable, pick a spot on the rim of the navel. Please remain on the rim, not inside the navel. Working inside the navel is too central, too intimate, and too intense.

Now, with your fingers, feel the quality of the skin and what's underneath it. Without lifting your fingers, make slow, rhythmic circles. After you have felt and nurtured that spot with at least several rotations, move slightly clockwise to another point on the navel rim. (Clockwise means moving toward your left hip.) Finger-circle at this new spot, gently, slowly, *while breathing into your belly.*

Move on until you have covered the entire rim of the navel. Be sensitive to any sensations of tension or areas of discomfort. Work those areas a bit more, gently, and with breath. I invite you to withhold judgement for now and to just ask yourself what it feels like. Check around the circumference of the navel again. Is the skin and what's underneath (only a half inch or so under the surface) starting to loosen up? Are there any changes?

Why You Work the Navel

This technique, simple as it may seem, can be profoundly relaxing. When done with gentle breathing, it connects you to your center in a very real sense, starting a process that will immediately begin to release tension.

How does it work? Some like to call the navel the original scar. But I like to think of it as the artifact, an imprint, if you will, of the bridge that once existed between you and your mother. Across this bridge you received nutrients and expelled waste. It's helpful to imagine that your entire body developed as an extension from this pathway, growing from your navel outward.

Embryologists observe a curious phenomenon. A fetus develops anatomical features at different rates and locales, but as each feature organizes interdependently, they remain linked to one another via the connective tissue. This connective tissue is really an interlocking web that holds various parts—the brain, the heart, the gut—together while the separate complex systems grow. That web of fascia of course still abides within us, and it would make sense that this web begins and ends at the navel.

If you regard the navel as the nexus of the fascial system, you can understand how you can affect a change throughout the entire body by bringing awareness to it via conscious breath and touch.

So with this technique, you are going to take advantage of this fundamental feature of centrality. By making contact and gently stimulating the skin and muscle that forms the navel, you encourage the entire body to relax.

If you were to do this one technique consistently (five minutes in the morning and evening) you could go a long way toward freeing up the entire body. When tension at the surface of the navel, on the skin, is released, there will be space for the underlying tension to travel through the many pathways of the web and up to the navel. This happy state of affairs would come about because you would be addressing new stress and toxicity before they had a chance to settle into the tissues of the body. That's a pretty advanced state of being, and you can keep that in mind for the long run. But for now, let's get rid of all the tension that has settled in over the years and that is making you tight.

I use this technique when I'm feeling uncomfortable after a less than optimal meal or to encourage a good bowel movement in the morning. It's also good for ridding myself of the previous day's stress, to set the pace of the new day, so that I can face whatever comes up with a relaxed body.

EXPLORING THE ABDOMINAL SURFACE WITH THE CAT'S PAWS TOUCH

Lie upon your back with your knees bent. Now you are going to use both hands, and you can employ two or more fingers, as many as is comfortable. Work your way out from the navel rim, touching, circling, massaging, and feeling: assessing the skin. First work a wider circle around the navel, then a yet wider circle, and then just move around at random, wherever your fingers want to go. Cover the entire abdomen from the bottom of the rib cage to the top of the hips and pubis.

Do not dig deep. Limit your touch to the surface of the skin and slightly underneath. Assess the quality of the skin, feeling for places that are tight, more sensitive than others, and for knots and tangles. You may encounter areas underneath the skin that feel like gravel, or even rocks. (Probably, that's the bound-up fascia surrounding your small intestine!) Is your skin damp, hot, watery, numb, or any combinations of these? What does it resemble: concrete, tofu, a bruise? Whatever it feels like, don't try to understand it right now, and especially don't judge it. Just feel.

Remember to keep breathing throughout the exercise. If you find a numb or uncomfortable place, continue to touch it for a bit, work at its edges, and try to focus your breath there. The time you take to explore will pay off in the future. Familiarize yourself with areas you may not have felt or breathed into for a very long time.

Once you have covered the entire abdomen, go over it again with both hands, massaging, alternating the hands rhythmically. Think of how a cat climbs on your lap and kneads it. This kneading action is what we will call "Cat's Paws." Do it in the same indescribably yummy way that a cat does it, strictly for the pleasure of it. It's a manipulation, but it's not poking or pushing, or done too rapidly; it's just right. And keep breathing.

Why You Work the Skin

The point of this exercise is to familiarize yourself with the shape, quality, and general terrain of the entire belly, to find out where the places of tension are, and where you have difficulty breathing or feeling. You might discover that there are lines of tension leading back from each sore area on the surface of the abdomen to a point of origin on the navel rim.

By working the entire surface of the abdomen you are preparing for deeper work. You can't expect to penetrate further if the surface is rigid and protecting against invasive touch. I guess you could try to force your way in, but I guarantee you it won't be at all pleasurable. (Isn't it uncomfortable when a massage therapist tries to delve in and applies too much pressure, without your body having time to adjust?) And I can promise you that it won't be very effective. The body is very good at resisting and evading what it isn't ready for. You have to coax it to truly relax and trust the process of healing. So it is absolutely vital that you go lightly, patiently, layer by layer. Otherwise, you will only create more tension.

When you gently stimulate the skin you are accessing and transmitting subtle messages. The nerves permeating the skin hold information about the level of stress and internal chemical and emotional states. This information is transmitted to the highly sensitive tips of the fingers and onward to areas of the brain where it is processed unconsciously or otherwise. With gentle touch you create an additional circuit of communication between the body and brain, but if you try to push beneath the outer layer of skin, or touch without breath and relaxed awareness, you will break this circuit (fig. 3.3).

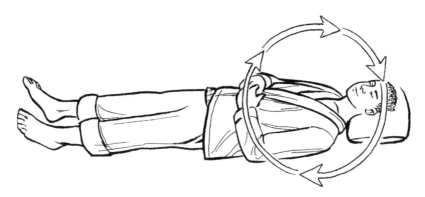

3.3. The circuit of healing. The circuit of healing runs from the skin through the fingertips to the brain, from the brain back to the viscera, and out to the skin again.

This feedback system, activated by delicate touch, has incredible healing power. This is not commonly known; it is one of the secrets of the healing arts and is the essence of my philosophy, so it's worth repeating: Delicate touch, combined with complete presence and unobtrusive listening, is far more effective than heavy-handedness. After all, isn't it the kind of touch you crave? Why wait for others to do it for you? Why not learn to open to it and give it to yourself right now?

LYMPH PUMPING

After you have softened the navel and worked the surface of the abdomen, you are ready to go a little deeper. Work at a place to the side of the navel, about the width of four fingers away. This is where there are natural, vertical creases on each side of the torso.

At this place you can dip in deeper and stimulate the abdominal lymph nodes. Use both hands, alternating in the same Cat's Paws motion that you used before. This should be very relaxing and stimulating at the same time. Be sure to breathe while you do this. You will know if you are too close to the navel because it will hurt and you won't be able to sink in very far. Likewise, if you are too far out from the navel it will be too sensitive, painful, or ticklish. That means you are aiming too wide. You will be able to sink, without pushing, approximately two to three inches deep, depending on your level of tension. Do this alternating, pumping action for about one complete minute.

Why You Pump the Lymph

Just below the surface abdominal muscles, the belly is literally covered with lymph tissue, and with the Cat's Paws technique, you stimulated it into action. The fluid in the lymph contains waste products from all the cells of the body. When it is stimulated, it travels toward the lymph nodes (places where there are masses of lymph tissue) that are deep within the abdomen. Within the nodes, the fluid is filtered of wastes. The practice of lymph pumping encourages this filtration process.

A NOTE ON ANATOMY AND PHYSIOLOGY

In my practice, I call these techniques "Unwinding," because they are very simple and natural exercises; you don't need to be an anatomist to gain benefit from them. With this and all the following techniques, when I direct you to touch a certain area, you do not have to do so with textbook precision.

In this book, I am purposely refraining from detailed anatomical description or complicated explanations of physiological function. My descriptions are simplified and may sound more poetic than scientific. I want to direct you to what you need to do in order for you to get better.

However, don't let my loose terminology throw you off. I want to keep it simple so that you can understand what to do and why you are doing it. If you want to learn more, there are wonderful books written on these vast subjects for the curious nonspecialist. But I don't want you to get hung up or overwhelmed with a monumental mass of abstract knowledge. Instead, I want you to engage with your body, learning what you need to learn as you go along.

If you want to delve further into anatomy and physiology, and I think it's important to do so the more you heal, I certainly encourage you to read more. As a caution though, it's my experience that clients who do know something of anatomy and physiology—but who are stressed or have trouble staying grounded—can sometimes let their knowledge get in the way. While working with yourself, instead of thinking too much, I invite you to feel.

So for right now, it's enough to know that lymph tissue filters the waste products of your cells. The only thing that gets the process going is movement. That is why you feel so sluggish when you don't move or exercise each day. The waste product just sits there, weighing you down, waiting to be moved. Before you can work on specific organs, you need to encourage movement, to get the waste moving toward the filtering stations of the abdominal lymph nodes and processed out of the belly.

JOAN'S STORY

I was introduced to my navel when I least expected it. I was so wrapped up in my busy life that I never expected to discover something so simple and yet so profound. The wonder of that experience was like a miracle to me. I consider the knowledge I gained from it invaluable.

My life was so full, I was always very busy achieving; twenty years as a film and television producer, a law school student, an MA program. All of this was exciting but I was—well there's no other way to describe it—unconscious. I was "Miss Type-A," marching blindly ahead, equating the mere achievement of goals with success in life.

Throughout my film career I was always bothered by stomach pain during productions. I took all the problems, all the crises, all the creative challenges, and held them tightly in my body. The funniest part of it was that I was famous for being the steady, stable caregiver. I soothed and calmed some of the most well-known television and film stars of that time. I was in great demand because everyone felt they were in good hands. They were right. Only *I* wasn't in my own good hands.

My wakeup call came when I was charging on to a new life as a lawyer in San Francisco. But I never saw San Francisco! Instead, I spent months cringing in the corner of my room, in pain, and crying a lot. I also gained a lot of weight. I finally realized my body was talking to me in a big way, but I didn't know what it was trying to tell me. I sought help.

Unwinding introduced me to my navel in a gradual way. It helped me work through the pain by bringing me to calmly accept my body's voice. Once I did that, the pain stopped! Through deep breathing and slow, gentle massage, my real self began to emerge.

But I wasn't finished learning the hard lessons of life yet. Two years later, I returned to the art world and produced a large-scale stage performance in Toronto. Back to the same pattern of caring for others in crises, ignoring my own problems, exerting a calming influence on everyone around me. This time it wasn't my stomach that reacted. I had a stroke!

Lying flat on my back, with fluids dripping into me from an intravenous injection, a cast on my leg from a recent tennis accident, I had never felt so helpless or inadequate. I asked myself what could I do. Was there a magic answer to my misery? Then I remembered what I had heard during one of my Unwinding sessions: "Be with yourself, unwind, and be okay with that." I didn't like that at all! But I started up my practice of Unwinding again and I slowly healed. I realize now that is exactly what needed to happen. I needed to be with myself, to understand and love myself with great compassion, and take the time to not do anything else.

After recovering from the stroke, I returned to San Francisco and received more training in Unwinding. This time, though, because of my struggles, I was blessed with a newfound awareness, experienced while breathing into my rib cage completely, expanding my breath to fill all the places of unconsciousness that felt like holes inside me. I could feel the power of vital energy flowing through me as I breathed not only in front but also through my back, sides, and entire chest. I have created a wonderfully open, expansive sanctuary within my body, where I am protected, supported, and encouraged. I travel there often.

Because of weight issues, paying attention to my navel used to be hard for me, but amazingly, the more I gently feel and acknowledge the tightness and blockages, the more I lose weight! My digestive system calmed down, so food is used, not stored as fat. Now there are no longer physical obstructions or self-deprecating attitudes standing between my awareness and my body. I realize that for me Unwinding is really about learning how to digest: how to digest emotions, how to digest sorrow and grief, how to digest life. I also realize that when I digest well, I clear all the clutter around me and really see who I am and my inborn potential. It is an incredibly empowering experience. The introduction to my navel led me to myself, to connections to my own birth and growth, and especially to the wonder and magic of life.

WHEN SHOULD I PRACTICE UNWINDING AND HOW MUCH SHOULD I DO AT A TIME?

There are two ways to look at this. The initial approach is going to be different from what comes later, after you have understood what it is all about.

The best way to learn a hands-on technique of any kind is to concentrate on it exclusively, without mixing it up with all the other activities you are participating in concurrently. So when you do Unwinding, keep it simple—just do Unwinding.

There is a principle in the healing arts that I find works very well. If you do something for thirty days—actually do it, not read about it—you will most likely experience self-evident, beneficial change. If you don't get any results after this period of honest effort, then that modality is not for you at this time. If you practiced Unwinding for even ten minutes each morning for thirty days, I would be very surprised if you did not recognize significant change.

I present Unwinding in simple steps to work through consecutively. In this way you will know you are making progress without feeling that you have to rush ahead and do it all at once. Ideally you would want to take your time, reviewing each step before moving on. You can read this book in a two-hour sitting, but the information is organized so that you can use it like a workbook. Practice each step as time permits. Refer back for periodic review to obtain additional insights.

I say practice for ten minutes, but you can work up to an hour if you want, but no more than that. I say each morning because I find that if any private work doesn't get done before the business of the day starts, it will most likely not get done. (And we are all busy, aren't we?) Unwinding gets the day started on the right foot, digestively and emotionally, and clears out any stagnancy from the previous night's sleep.

Continue Unwinding through the successive steps on a disciplined path until you think you really understand it. Thoroughly review any time in your life when you are challenged with difficulties. That's the ideal. Apart from that, I sincerely hope you go through the sequence any which way you can fit the work in.

After thoroughly learning Unwinding for the first time I encourage you to creatively adapt it to the rest of your life. Each person is so different that I can only give some examples of the way I use Unwinding.

When I have overworked or overplayed and as a result I am fatigued, thinking too much, or can't sleep, I find a place to lie down, breathe, touch my belly, and do nothing else. I do it wherever I happen to be, whether at the beach, a friend's house, or visiting family. Please take time out for yourself. It is not as if you will be arrested for spending ten to twenty minutes in privacy.

I often unwind in between clients. I do it to settle my energy, to make separation from the last client, and to clear my mind for the next. You don't have to be a therapist to do this; a few moments by yourself can make the noise of the day into rhythmic music, a music that lets you waltz through your workday. (Or salsa, if you prefer.) You can take what seems like an overwhelming onslaught of responsibilities and chop it up into small bites by taking a few short Unwinding breaks. I realize you can't lie on the office floor, unless, of course, you are the boss. That's where the standing posture comes in handy (chapter 7). Once you have learned the techniques, you can do everything standing. Unwinding can also be done sitting, although it takes a high level of concentrated relaxation.

I unwind before bed if I've had a late or heavy meal. Why allow my precious sleep (when regeneration occurs) to be disrupted by indigestion?

I do a lot of thorough, deep Unwinding on vacation. This is how I expand it, discovering new things. On vacation I exchange sessions with Stephen—we work on each other—but this is more in the line of an enhanced communication art. You have to be careful working with a spouse or a friend; keep it fun. Working on the belly can be tricky, and it's not normally part of a romantic relationship. As I said, it is a special communication tool, perhaps to be part of another book. I'll only say here, keep it fun and don't talk! Just breathe and touch. Discussion, interpretation, or commentary is not part of it. Healing is something a loved one has to first take in hand voluntarily.

This breathing and touching without talking takes a huge amount of discipline, though. Please concentrate on Unwinding yourself first. Spouses, lovers, friends, and family can unconsciously (or not) derail the process. Remember that inept breathing and unhealthy patterns are socially derived phenomena. Do not allow your practice to be subject to negotiation or influenced by the ever-present habit of comparison to others. Most activities in life involve a bargaining process between you and others, but personal health should remain a personal matter. Mark out a place and time for yourself and give yourself this gift. You deserve it.

4

Intermediate Steps in Unwinding—
Lateral Breathing and Elimination

This new exercise is deceptively short and simple. But please don't underestimate the effect it can have on your overall well-being. It does not take much time to perform, but the more times you practice, the better you unwind. You are going to expand the reach of the breath into areas that are frozen up in most people. You will be allowing more space for blood and oxygen to feed important organs and connective structures within the belly. Also, with this exercise you will discover why it is important to put your knees up. If you try it with the knees down, the muscles of the body are engaged in such a way that the diaphragm does not have the freedom to expand its range.

LATERAL BREATHING

Lying on a flat surface with your knees up, place your left hand on the side of the belly, covering the left ribs. Hold firmly, offering some resistance. Begin to breathe down into the belly as in Belly Breathing, but this time direct your breath to expand the left side out, laterally. The hand cups the ribs, not fighting or constricting the outward movement, but to give enough pressure to determine if, and how much, you are able to breathe into and fill that area (fig. 4.1). You don't want to feel your chest and rib muscles flexing just to give the sensation of movement. You want to feel the relaxed muscles of the ribs rising and falling due only to the internal pressure of the breath.

Since this is a new place to breathe (most likely it has been neglected for quite a long time), it may require lots of practice and patience. You want your hand on the ribs to give something for the breath to work against. It is an exercise for the breath to fill space as the muscles and ribs expand. Anyone can flex the abdominal muscles and produce movement to the side without breathing, awkward as it may be. Try it the wrong way once so that your inner sense can distinguish the not so obvious difference between contracted "breathing" and relaxed lateral expansion. Then try it again with the breath, the hand cupped firmly on the side of the relaxed but moving ribs.

Now with the right hand, try it on the right rib cage (fig. 4.2). Be sure to give yourself plenty of time to practice on this side, becoming more and more refined in feeling the expansion rather than forcing the movement.

You will discover that the key to getting the ribs to expand laterally in a relaxed fashion is to take in more air. The commonplace way of breathing with short, quick, contracting gasps does not do the job.

After feeling improvement on both sides, combine the two together. Now you really need to take in a lot of air! Keep practicing, holding the left and right ribs, directing the breath into both sides, filling up the belly sideways (fig. 4.3). Notice how much play you get in the rib cage, which side is tighter, and if it is difficult to remain calm while practicing. Don't interpret this information. Just note how it is to breathe laterally.

As a general guideline, I recommend that within each session you practice Lateral Breathing at least ten times on the left, ten times on the right, and then ten times together.

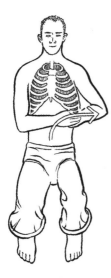 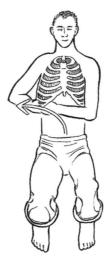 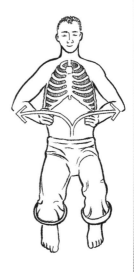

4.1. Lateral breathing—left side. Breath from the belly fills up and then expands laterally into the left rib cage.

4.2. Lateral breathing—right side. Breath from the belly fills up and then expands laterally into the right rib cage.

4.3. Full lateral breathing. Breath from the belly expands both sides of the rib cage simultaneously.

Understanding Lateral Breathing

The diaphragm—the muscle you use to breathe in a natural, relaxed way—is attached to the rib cage. When you expand the freedom of breath and movement of the rib cage you loosen and enliven the diaphragm. The diaphragm is not a flat surface but dome-shaped, and so the sides cover and connect to a larger portion of the viscera than does the center area of the muscle (fig. 4.4). If you were to breathe only into the frontal plane of the belly you would not be tapping into the full power of breathing—not even by half! Probably it has been a very long time (perhaps since infancy) since you have used this greater portion of the diaphragm. Like any other muscle within the body, if not utilized, it will soon weaken and eventually atrophy. But happily, it is also like other muscles in that it will come back to life. When it is exercised, when it is moved, it literally regenerates itself!

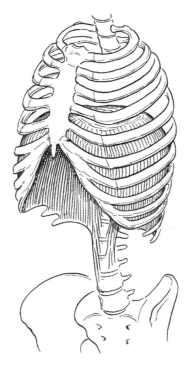

4.4. The shape of the relaxed, healthy diaphragm.

Lateral Breathing is also beneficial for the internal organs. Tucked up under the rib cage on the left side are the stomach, spleen, and pancreas. Under the center and right reside the gallbladder and liver. That's a lot of tissue in not a lot of space, and a tight and immovable rib cage will constrict and choke it. These organs perform countless functions of digestion and metabolism. The number of diseases connected with impaired functions of these vital organs is also countless, so you want to provide a full, smooth, continuous, oxygen-rich blood supply to them.

You also want to stay connected to these organs in a feeling state so that you are aware of any dysfunction, long before symptoms of disease begin to manifest. Generally, the body changes to a state of imbalance first in the internal organs, and it is difficult to know if anything is amiss on the inside—the invisible part of the body. When you develop a practice of full breathing, with awareness, you will have a much better likelihood of feeling something awry within the system. The initial stage of imbalance is critical because that is when you can adjust in ways the body is signaling for. As you know, the bulk of the present-day medical system is designed to counteract the process of disease *after* serious symptoms manifest. Lateral Breathing, along with all of Unwinding, is simply Preventative Medicine 101.

There is something curious about the sides of the trunk. It seems to be the easiest and most common area to disconnect from, to develop the habit of not feeling anything. This happens in spite of the fact that we know it is a very personal part of the body. We are so used to having our arms down by our sides to guard from outside invasion that we rarely notice how personal it is. But think how vulnerable you feel when you put your arms up in the company of strangers. You get that awkward, silly, exposed, or submissive feeling, and it happens for a reason. Your body is wisely cautious about exposing those vital organs. Those funny ticklish areas on the sides of the belly are there to monitor how the organs are doing internally and to register when those organs are exposed to external forces.

Loosening up the sides of the trunk can have a dramatic effect on the mobility of the entire upper body. In my experience anyone bothered with a tight chest, cramped shoulders, and stiff neck invariably also has a restricted rib cage. This is why any stretching routine worth its salt (and time), for any sports activity, includes side-bends. One of the reasons a side-bend can be so difficult at first, yet feel so good when it is done for more than a few quick seconds, is because it allows room for the organs to release pent up, stale energy, letting it flow out from the area. When the trunk muscles stretch and relax, the muscle and bones in the upper body begin to realign into their proper positions.

Enhanced lateral movement in the rib cage also allows the body more options in overall movement, and a wider repertoire in feeling, thoughts, and body language expressed by that movement (fig. 4.5). Most people are pretty much locked into focusing on the frontal plane, struggling to constantly "move forward," "look ahead," and "face problems." Going backward is a bad thing,

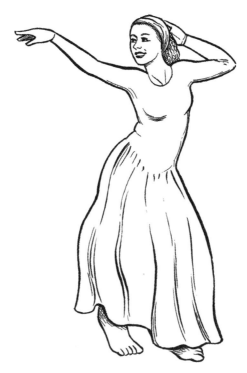

4.5. Enhanced lateral movement. Enhanced lateral movement of the diaphragm and rib cage gives more options in expressive movement and body language.

we've all been told, and when we think we are not getting anywhere we say we are "going around in circles." Moving, being aware, and thinking laterally? Well, that sounds downright suspicious. What are we left with, then, with this kind of attitude, with this limited approach, of always wanting to face and move (and breathe) forward into one-dimensional space? Barrel chests, cramped shoulders, and stiff necks! Those are the most common symptoms of a rigid, inhibited form of expression. Nature's way, though, is not linear, but uses the indirect path. Anything natural, including your body, grows and moves (and heals!) in circles and arcs and waves and spirals and in many patterns at once. Lateral Breathing, in a very subtle yet profound way, can help your body and mind move in a variety of ways, in accordance with the three-dimensional, curved structure of the body, within the squiggly shape of nature.

CONNECTING TO THE
LARGE INTESTINE (COLON)

Read through this step a few times before performing it, because it's a bit complicated. Once you get it, though, it makes perfect sense. You will be working the outside edges of the surface of the belly, from left to right, but moving up the circle in stages, connecting each new segment to the ones previously worked. Rest assured it's the most involved technique of Unwinding; everything after this is easy. It's a good idea to have someone read out the directions as you find the positions and sequence of the technique. However, if you prefer, there are audio and video options available on our website.

Lying on a comfortable surface with knees up, find the soft place between the bottom of the left rib cage and the top of the bony part of the left hip. This will be as far to the left side of the belly as you can get without working in horizontally from the side. With both hands, use the Cat's Paws technique with alternating hands as you did before. As you gently loosen this area, encourage relaxation in the direction of the pubis, scooping slightly downwards. But don't go as far as the area below the navel. Work the soft space between the rib cage and hip. Keep your shoulders and elbows relaxed, left elbow on the floor, if you can reach, and right arm resting on the belly. Try to keep your wrists and fingers soft. If you work with tense muscles or are holding up your elbows, you will quickly tire.

After you have loosened this area, move to a central place, between the center of the rib cage and the navel. Massage this area until it feels decongested. Now, instead of lifting the hands to move to the next place, work your way over, cat's-pawing all the while, to the left side again to where you were before, and loosen that even more, encouraging a downward flow.

Now, lift your hands and place them below the lowest rib on the right side, and cat's-paw there. Be a bit more specific here than on the left side, but you don't have to work down to the right hip. After you have loosened below the right rib, connect from there, across the center, and around the left side down to the left hip again.

Now the fourth and final area: Place your hands at a spot halfway between your right hip and navel and cat's-paw again until you feel it loosen, slowly and gently. Then go ahead and connect all the areas, from the lower right side, up to the right rib, across, down the left side and then encourage movement toward the left hip and pelvis. Go over the entire right to left pathway as many times as necessary to loosen and encourage movement.

This technique may not be pleasant at first. In fact, it can feel downright uncomfortable, particularly on the right side. But as you continue to unwind it should become less obstructed. You will know how much to work and when to stop in each session. If you experience pain, don't work directly on that spot. Work the areas around it, making space for the pain to disperse into. Work longer with the unobstructed areas. Be gentle and compassionate with yourself and remember to breathe.

Understanding the Colon

After the small intestine has absorbed all it can from food, the remaining material (watch out folks, this gets graphic) is squirted through the ileocecal valve into the colon. This valve (pronounced "ee-lee-o-see-kel") was that spot on the lower right side of the belly that might have felt sore. Within the colon, the body extracts vital minerals and as much water as it can, and thereby forms the feces, which are shunted to the rectum and expelled from the body. The pathway of the colon, in general terms, is from the right side, upward, across, down the left side, curving toward the midline, and continuing to the rectum.

When you work with the colon in the order described above, you are first clearing the end of the pathway before encouraging movement at the beginning of the pathway. You don't want to make the mistake of trying to force wastes to move where there is no space for them to go because it won't work and will feel very uncomfortable.

The body needs time to extract water and minerals and to form the feces, so the colon is long (about five feet). For these reasons it is situated within the belly in an interesting shape. Material passing through it has to defy gravity while coming up the right side, then it makes a sharp turn, runs across the belly, makes a loop behind the stomach, makes another sharp turn to go down the left side, and finally makes an S-curve to pass into the rectum (fig. 4.6). To get the job done the colon uses its own natural form of Cat's Paws movement, alternating between contraction and release, and you are kindly helping it out.

There are two ligaments (one on each side of the rib cage) that hold up the section of the colon that runs across the belly. These ligaments are important because they connect to that magical breathing muscle, the diaphragm. When you become physically stressed or emotionally upset, and breathe up into your chest instead of downward and laterally in the lower rib cage, these ligaments become tightly constricted. The turns and bends of the colon (the flexures) will become restricted, or even twisted about. Then it is going to be very difficult to have smooth elimination. This technique softens and strengthens these ligaments and unravels any knots in the colon.

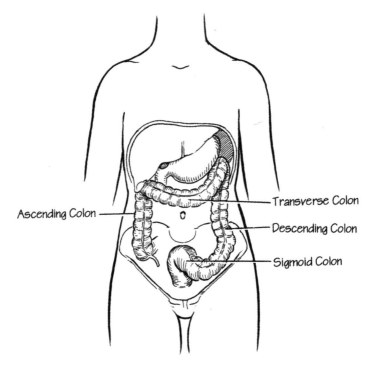

Ascending Colon

Transverse Colon

Descending Colon

Sigmoid Colon

4.6. The shape of the relaxed, healthy colon.

The colon is an exquisitely sensitive organ. It reacts to all manner of stress, physical and emotional. For instance, think how immediately the colon reacts to a situation of extreme fear. Releasing tension from contracted ligaments and soothing and relaxing the colon can be emotionally stirring work for anyone who has suppressed any kind of emotion, which includes just about everyone.

Breathing naturally with the diaphragm activates the nerves in all the organs of the belly. This is how our inner awareness is connected in an exact and amazingly specific manner to every impulse from the acutely mood-sensitive colon. If something is not sitting right, physically or emotionally, the colon is privy to that information. Breathing with the full diaphragm while stimulating the colon is one of the most precise means of connecting to how you feel in the moment and to how you have dealt with past stresses.

You can tap into the energy of the colon to beneficially modulate your present internal state and improve your coping strategy.

BOWEL MOVEMENTS AND STOOLS

Now that you have worked on the large intestine I think I should share my thoughts on how important it is for you to keep an eye on the end result of all that good eating you've been doing. Even in our day and age, where it seems people can talk about anything, they still don't like to talk about bowel movements and stools. Maybe it's not the best conversation at a cocktail party, but it certainly is an appropriate topic with anyone who is advising you about your health. It is also vitally important for you to develop an ongoing, personal chat with your body. Keep in mind that elimination is one of the primary means your body has to communicate with you, and hopefully, you get a daily report!

I have discovered in my teaching and practice that most people have a real aversion to glancing back at their stools before flushing. If you've got the heebie-jeebies just reading this, please refer to one of my favorite books listed in the resources. It is a book for children of all ages entitled: *Everyone Poops.* If you're uncomfortable with the idea of taking an interest in this subject, take it as a sign that all may not be well with you. In my experience, every healthy person that I've ever met knows what comes out of her bowels and uses that information to stay on a healthy track.

Your stool is the product of what you have eaten and what your digestive system has done with your food. This depends on to what degree the food was digestible (if at all) and the existing state of tension and stress within your belly before the meal. You must also consider the stress the meal itself caused, if you were chewing thoroughly, and what you might have been doing during and directly after the meal. Were you arguing, rushing, or working? Were you eating while driving, *and* halfway to road rage? The state of tension during elimination is also important. Were you rushing, pushing, worrying or ... reading? All these factors together produce the stool that tells you how you are doing, both digestively and stress-wise.

Enough philosophy! I have been asked with much vexation many times: "What is my stool supposed to look like?" Since everyone is so different and individual, I can only answer in general terms. Further, if I can digress again, I'm not suggesting that you can diagnose disease in this way. You can discover *dis-ease,* to know when things aren't working right, and taking a look at your stool is one way to catch developments before you get sick—but only if you're willing to look. I think of the bowel and its movements as the original biofeedback machine that helps us monitor our health. But keep in mind that even with the guidelines that follow, your body is constantly passing through various, natural cycles that could affect the quality of bowel movements.

So what are our bowel movements supposed to be like? Well, first of all, if you see blood I suggest you see a medical doctor for testing. Very black stools may indicate bleeding in the upper regions of the digestive system and may also require a test. Pale or clay-colored stools could mean your liver or gallbladder is not producing enough bile, or is otherwise out of sorts and needs attention. A functional medicine practitioner can offer a holistic approach to treatment here, rather than pressuring you to jump to a surgical solution.

Food particles in the stool beg that you reconfigure your diet, food combining, and exercise strategies. (Of course you will have to account for roughage or fiber, which I do hope you include in your diet.) Consistently bad smelling poop tells you that you may not have the right bacterial balance in the colon. This calls for a change in diet to see which food or foods are not being digested, or, if you have tried that with no success, a comprehensive stool analysis.

When you make a lifestyle change, you will see almost immediate changes in poop; I guarantee it. What you are working toward are brown poops in large, long, unbroken banana-like shapes. Not balls, or pieces that are ribbed and pocketed—you are after smooth surfaces. (All shades of brown are okay, but the color will vary somewhat, in tandem with your diet.) Pencil-thin or ribbon-like stools could indicate a polyp or growth in the colon that has narrowed the passage. The shape is basically determined by the shape of the lower segment of the colon, which changes due to emotional tension and obstruction.

Of course, constipation is not good. Straining and difficulty is not a good sign either. It is important to have at least one good movement per day, yet this can vary from person to person. If you are eliminating less often than once per day, check your daily intake of water and fiber.

I remember one woman who told me that upon waking up each day, she was so immediately and busily involved with getting her children, her husband, and herself up, fed, and off to school and work, that she delayed answering the natural urge. When she finally had time for the morning bowel movement the opportunity was lost. That part of her body function, unheeded, efficiently shut down until … well the entire workday was done and the children's homework completed and they were fed and put to bed, and hubby attended to … well, maybe then. She asked me if this qualified as constipation.

The short answer is yes. But you can see there is no easy cause and effect going on with poop. I can't show you a chart with a simple formula that says if you have this it's because of that. Constipation is often caused by poor diet, but it can also occur from a variety of interconnected causes. Bodily function, like life itself, happens in the context of everything else that's happening. Once you get the idea that your stools are important, you can take the lead and figure out the how and why of your poop and your body.

Diarrhea is not a good sign and calls for drastic behavior changes. You may want to track carefully what you are eating so that you can figure out what brings on the reaction. Parasites, viruses, or too much caffeine can also cause diarrhea. If diarrhea continues to be persistent, I encourage you to consult with your health care provider.

Alternating bouts of constipation and diarrhea (irritable bowel syndrome) tells a jumbled story that may include diet, allergies, laxative abuse, chronic worry, and chaotic relationships. Or it might be due to the side effects of medication and supplements, or an overconsumption of sugar and alcohol. It will take time and effort to unravel this story, but pick one element to work on and start there. But while you do your part, irritable bowel syndrome calls for a full review with someone versed in functional medicine, because it could very well signal an imbalance in the gut flora or an allergy or sensitivity to a particular food or foods.

And there are other forms of intestinal imbalance that cause irritation and inflammation. These can include an inability to digest some forms of proteins, fats or carbohydrates, low acid or an overgrowth *of Helicobacter pylori in* the stomach. These sometimes go hand in hand with bacterial overgrowth in the small or large intestine. Again, conducting a comprehensive stool analysis will serve you well if you are hounded by chronic digestive problems.

It may sound strange, but in my practice I've met many people who have gotten so used to the two conditions of constipation and diarrhea that they consider them normal or not worthy of serious thought. I know how busy a person can get, wrapped up in the rush of so many things to do. But now you know that diarrhea, constipation, or continuous switching from one to the other is not normal and needs your attention. Your body is trying to tell you something.

Loose stools have too much water or mucus. They don't hold together, but break apart. If mucus is in your stool it could be another indication of less than optimal food or poor food combination, dehydration, or inflammation in the bowel. Mucus is a natural lining in your bowel that needs to stay put because it lubricates and makes for happy elimination. I say "happy" seriously. If there is not a certain pleasure with elimination, you should consider making adjustments to your diet or exercise, check in on your stress levels, and, of course, unwind your belly. Elimination is a vital part of your daily routine, and you can think of it as one among the other skills of restoring your gut health.

We've made it through our confidential poop talk. Congratulations! Now, I'm not suggesting that you become obsessed with your stool. I do suggest you respect your bowel movements as a very real representation of the underbelly of life, the shadow: all the stuff we'd rather bury out of sight and ignore. As you know, there's no such thing as a one-sided coin. So why pretend there's no flip side to eating? Being conscious of both what's being taken in and what's coming out is a real skill of healthy living, and I hope you develop this skill with the perfect blend of seriousness and lightheartedness that it deserves.

MARGUERITE'S STORY

When I was in my late twenties, one of my main concerns was to remain as thin as possible. Now that I can look back on it with equanimity, I can say that my behavior was quite erratic. Some days I would maintain a rigorous diet, consisting of only one meal per day of fruits and salad. On other days I managed to not obsess, and I ate anything that came my way. And some days, I have to admit, I would binge. This fluctuating diet, coupled with the other usual stresses of life, brought me to a state in which my body temperature was uncomfortably hot, and most of the time I was severely constipated. I think I went on like this for five to seven years.

I knew my digestion was poor because everything in and outside of me began to feel heavy, as if life were slowing me down. I knew I had a lot of energy, but could never tap into it. I sought out massage therapy because my body usually felt like it had been beaten up and needed to be soothed. A friend of mine passed on a brochure describing Unwinding. Two words stood out: "digestion" and "metabolism." I was sold.

The first session was uncomfortable. It wasn't painful, but touching around the navel felt odd and unnatural. I felt stiff muscles around my navel that I had never felt before.

Soon I learned to breathe naturally by watching my belly go up and down as I practiced.

Now I look forward to rubbing my own belly. Whenever I feel pain or constipation I practice the technique of starting under the left rib cage and following the path of the large intestine. I can get my digestion and metabolism to run more smoothly just by breathing and touching. Every time I feel panicky and out of control, I hear a little voice in my head saying: "Breathe!"

All this is wonderful, and yet I made another unexpected discovery. Unwinding can definitely be an emotional experience. During the first few sessions I felt like bawling. At the time, I was contemplating divorce—that was part of why I felt so emotional—but I learned how old patterns of tension in the center influence how we feel in the present moment. This rang true for me. As I continued to loosen up with my self-massage sessions, I felt the whole bag of past emotional garbage that I was carrying around unload into the accepting earth, where it belonged, where it could be recycled.

Another wonderful thing was that I began to feel more comfortable with my belly. I still wanted to maintain a good figure, but in a healthy way. This was because I was touching and relating to my belly; I wasn't sucking it in and hiding it, pretending it wasn't there. I could look at my own belly and even enjoy the sight of it. My motivation to stay thin is now in balance with the rest of my life.

HOW DOES UNWINDING DIFFER FROM OTHER SYSTEMS OF WORKING WITH THE BREATH AND THE VISCERA?

Unwinding is simple in philosophy and approach. It is about embracing simplicity. That doesn't mean it's superficial or easy, as you will see just as soon as you begin to practice.

A distinguishing feature of Unwinding is that the breathing is always gentle and practiced in stages. Take your time with it. Just like when you learn anything new, a slow and steady approach, a little bit each day, is better than the weekend warrior approach. In other words, the breathing is not meant to bring on an unmanageable hailstorm of memory and emotion. Also, the deep breathing exercises in Unwinding are exercises to do specifically during practice. They will eventually bring about healthy, natural breathing patterns done in a spontaneous fashion during the other times of your life. In your day-to-day life, you are welcome to keep the mouth closed (with a relaxed jaw, of course) on both inhale and exhale.

The touch techniques are very gentle. You work on yourself with a slow tempo. You're not pounding, bruising, or trying to get things done in a hurry. Unwinding is not designed for others to dig around in your guts doing the work for you, on their time schedule. You stay with your feeling and don't get hung up on a practitioner's or your own interpretation of your symptoms. Of course, a practitioner can be both knowledgeable and skilled, but if she understands her work thoroughly, she will lead you to the simple state of being quiet with yourself. At that point she will have the wisdom to back off and listen with you. If not, well, you can always relax, unwind, and embody at home. Use your skill to complement the "for-pay" therapies you receive. But this means you will have to be a self-starter as far as motivation goes.

The hardest thing to do in life is to keep it simple. As you learn more about yourself you will come to appreciate the complexity of the biology of the gut, the impact of nutrition, and the vitality of your emotions. But that doesn't mean you lose yourself. Recognize that you move and live in complexity, but ride through it all with serenity.

As my practice continues, I tend to touch more and more lightly. In fact, I don't consider Unwinding to be a form of massage therapy. Instead, it is a way *to embody.*

Embodiment means different things to different people, but to me it means simply sensing inside my body while maintaining awareness of the space around me. When we unwind, we're not necessarily trying to fix or do anything. Rather, we are meeting, in a quiet and open-minded way, what's already there, and then opening up to the possibility of our body finding a way to unravel tension with the least amount of effort. Sometimes I think of Unwinding as a kind of meditation, a meditation upon how you are doing, physically, in the present moment, and how you are feeling. But of course the word meditation can bring up unnecessary complications for some, so I prefer to think of Unwinding as a gentle exercise of exploration, done with compassion and curiosity. Nothing more, nothing less.

When I teach workshops, the students and I spend a lot of time doing exercises that resemble meditation, and when we work on ourselves (and sometimes each other) we do so with an open mind, with no goals. Considerations of healing or curing are put to the side and instead we practice listening—listening to silence, sensing stillness, and then hearing what's truly present in the body. In my audio and my video course, the intent is the same. I gently guide an exploration by listening and feeling, allowing the breath to find space in the body—space in which to unwind tension—and to sense the natural rhythms of pulsating life, however subtle, that resonate around you and within you.

Sometimes when I unwind myself, I don't touch at all. I sit or lie down and go inside—I won't say mentally, because that calls up the idea of picturing things. I go in with feeling. I feel the various tissues of my body, and I give them breath and space. The blood, the bones, the fascia, the nerves, and all the rest, are alive and resonant with…well, with being.

Anyone can do this if they breathe naturally and are still, not rushing or forcing anything. Anyone can learn to listen, to touch, and to be still, and anyone can develop an acute inner kinesthetic sense, a sense of body and of self. There is no such thing as a totally visual or auditory person. (The kinesthetic sense had to be there; otherwise you wouldn't have grown up to be a functioning adult.) And anyway, these various pathways of knowing are all of a piece. You have the neural network; the map that creates and interprets the territory of life is in the brain and in the body. And it is a soft-wired system; it can adapt, change, grow, and learn. It just takes sitting quietly and giving it a try.

And finally, I would add that Unwinding and a deeper embodiment practice can be a bridge for you. This bridge can lead to the development of the kind of holistic sensibility that will help you navigate the discomforts, the confusions, and the complexities that come with the nervous, hormonal, and other body-system dysfunctions connected with gut imbalances. This holistic sensibility can even guide you through the maze of dietary advice and the larger issues of the continuing deterioration in the quality of the food supply and in the environment.

The time you take now settling into a belly-centered wisdom will be well spent, something that will last you a lifetime.

5

Gut Matters

Before moving on to deeper breathing and more touch, I'd like to pause to once again caution against racing through the steps, and to address some important matters. These matters cannot be ignored if you desire to be comfortable enough in your body to become the primary guide in your healing journey.

A DEEPER UNDERSTANDING

Anyone who wishes to be fully embodied, in a belly-centered way, needs a deeper understanding of the digestive system and its connection to the rest of the body. I call these in-depth considerations "gut matters" because the entire body and the brain is affected by the health of the gut, and for any healing to take place that is more than the temporary suppression of symptoms, we must consistently return to deepen our understanding and appreciation of the belly. In other words, we must go from belly to guts!

In chapter 2, I outlined why I believe the belly is so important to your digestion, your emotion, and your movement, and why I consider these three aspects fundamental to health. But the belly can also be seen in a different light, for I believe the amazing biology of the digestive organs of the gut, the way these organs are intertwined and connected to each other and to the rest of the body, and the rich, natural environment in which they exist—all work together to maintain your health and your very being.

Over the last several decades, I have seen a disturbing trend in my practice. Although the people I see love to relax with me, rediscover their breath, and be guided to connect with an inner-body sense of themselves, many have difficulty going much further. This seems to be happening more often. No matter how much clients would like to make the changes they desire, they either still feel chained to the past or they bump up against new, vague, and even mysterious obstacles.

It is true that many of these obstacles are related to the ramped-up levels of stress in our lives. This stress is introduced into our systems by so many new vectors—financial strain, overwork, the overstimulation from exposure to computer-driven reality, a continuing degradation of the environment and food supply, a deteriorating health care system, and so much else. But it is also true that more and more people, no matter how well they are coping, are frustrated by challenges that are not being adequately addressed by the usual therapies, treatments, medications, and mind/body strategies.

In my current practice I am meeting many forthright and committed seekers who eat well, exercise vigorously, and devote a considerable amount of their time to relax and de-stress, yet they continue to be plagued with bothersome syndromes or—in one way or another—become frustrated in their search for the proverbial glow of health. Some are even devoted meditators but can't seem to embody unless they are *in meditation,* while others seem to be unable to connect socially or even to themselves, or find satisfaction and meaning in life.

All too often I have had to ask myself, "How can that be?" But as I continue to study and apply what I learn to my own healing, I keep making more discoveries. So I believe that if you find yourself at a plateau and not able to make further progress, you can surely benefit by seeing your belly in a new light and working with it in new ways.

First, let me say that I don't know all the answers, nor do I pretend to know the ultimate source of suffering in this universe. But I do know that you will be able to find many practical avenues of relief if you continue to search for solutions. Understanding your belly in a general way is wonderful, but considering it as all the juicy bits at the core of your daily life, as your guts, will motivate you to seek new therapeutic approaches. And that way, you will be able to continue the step-by-step process of restoring your gut health by going deeper into your body, finding and settling into a form of vibrant health that is perfectly suited to your life. After having gone deep into the unglamorous gut, you can reemerge into a perhaps more civilized, belly-centered life.

So together, let's explore more reasons why your belly—your gut—leads the way.

THE THREE TUBES OF THE EMBRYO

Soon after you were conceived, you quickly became a collection of rapidly dividing cells, floating in the fluid within your mother's womb and being nourished through the umbilicus. But then another miracle-like event occurred. The collection of cells elongated to form three streaks or lines, and although microscopically small, they were three-dimensional, tube-like shapes.

In a very general but nevertheless meaningful sense, these three tubes were creating the three principal organs of the body and their supporting structures. They developed into the three primary systems of your living body. These three streaks or tubes would later of course interact in extremely complex ways, and come to work in sync throughout your life, but they can be seen to have started out as distinct. In fact, it is helpful at times to think about them as three separate layers of the body. These three are the heart and the circulatory system, the brain and the nervous system, and the more primitive gut and gastrointestinal system.

I call the gastrointestinal system more primitive because it still is pretty much just a tube, beginning at the mouth and ending at the anus. Although amazingly complex, it doesn't have the branch pattern that we see in the circulatory or nervous systems, and, in a very general sense, its function can be understood as pretty straightforward. Food and liquid are ingested and, unless they are sensed as a poison and quickly repelled, move through the body from top to bottom. The tube kicks into gear as soon as eating or drinking is anticipated, and it will continue to do its thing until the ingested material is completely dealt with.

Digestion is basically a process whereby food and liquid are processed into smaller molecules so they can be carried through the very thin wall of the tube and into the circulatory system. Once through that thin wall, they are transported to the liver for sampling, storage, or elimination, or they are carried to the rest of the body via the blood in the circulatory system. What liquid is not used (and recycled in the colon) gets passed to the urinary system, and the part of food that is not digestible is eventually ejected from the end of the gut tube.

As I mentioned, most of the digestible food is ferried to the circulatory system for further transport, and all of this activity is moderated by the nervous system. So we have the three general, original tubes that first elongated in streak-like forms in the embryo, now working in tandem as three fully developed and integrated systems.

Detailed descriptions and discussions of these three systems fill countless volumes, but I've shared my very simplified vision to point to the fact that the gut tube—the more primitive and earthy—is the primary way, along with breathing, that we make contact with the outer environment.

This is important to keep in mind because we can be distracted by our central nervous system. When taking in so many impressions (light and sound and other vibrations, and so much more!) the brain is stimulated and the mind produces its panoply of fascinating representations. It does such a good job of this that we tend to forget that the outside world is also coming into our bodies each and every day in a much more primal way. We're so busy having the many ideas and thoughts that color life that it's easy to forget, and tempting to discount, the importance of the primary way we take in the outer world.

As we make this physical contact with the outer world, taking in oxygen, liquid, and food we are also ingesting a fair amount of microorganisms. In fact we are taking in entire colonies of microorganisms, comprised of hundreds of species. These are joining colonies that have already taken up residence within the primitive gut tube in the body. So when you eat and drink and breathe, you are merely adding to or replacing a community of microbiota that is already there.

These little guys, as I call them, were not there when you were a developing embryo (rare viral infections, aside). You were protected from them by the watery womb. These colonies of microbes first got in there when you made your very messy entrance to the outside environment, when you passed through the birth canal covered in mucus and other unglamorous fluids, when you took your first gasps of air, and when you took your first milky meal. The little guys were waiting for you, in the fluids that coat the birth canal, in the air, in the food, on the skin of your mother, on every surface in the room. Some of these microbiota immediately set up shop on every inch of your skin. Others took up residence in the mucosal lining of your gut tube, from mouth to anus.

Birth is a two-way street. When you were born, you entered and became part of the world, but at the same time the world entered and became part of you.

These little guys, otherwise known as your microbiota, were—and are—mostly bacteria. But there are also fungi (yeast), primitive single-celled organisms called archaea, protozoa, and "nonliving" viruses too.

Having colonies of bacteria on and inside of your body might strike you as a disaster, but before you make a dash for the shower or medicine cabinet, recall that having these colonies as part of you is perfectly natural. These various organisms coexist in complex communities, which means they compete for space and food, and ideally, keep one another in check. Fortunately, while doing so, they provide many benefits.

Let's also keep in mind that colonies of microbes inhabit—as far as we can tell—almost every environment, from the deep ocean vents to the sand at the beach, in the soil, and in the atmosphere. I believe that there are many more species of microbiota to be discovered than there are currently known, and as the planet goes through its inevitable cooling and warming stages, more species will evolve and some of them will no doubt be released from the vast permafrost that covers much of the northern latitudes. Microbes also exist on and inside the plants and animals we eat, and on every surface we touch.

My point is, that even if you'd like to be free of them, that's not going to be possible. And because they confer benefits, being cleansed of them would not be desirable. They confer benefits because we have evolved in tandem with them, and as we evolved, we came to depend upon their aid in digestion and so many more vital functions. So these colonies of microbes have been our allies, for better or for worse, as long as human beings have been around. Our very evolution took place, and continues to take place, in their presence. The body and its microbiota continue to evolve together in a symbiotic dance. We wouldn't be human without them, and we probably won't be able to evolve into better forms of ourselves without knowing more about them. So I think it behooves us to learn about them and to work with them to improve our health.

These colonies might be a collection of little guys, but they do add up. Although I haven't made a count myself, I've read that the number of cells of your microbiota outnumber the number of your somatic (body) cells by a factor of two to one. (Some scientists say it could be as much as three to one.) That makes for trillions of these little guys, and they can add up to weigh as much as three pounds, which is approximately the weight of your brain. So yes, they might be little, but they are many and, because the majority live inside of the primitive, gastrointestinal tube that is your gut, they carry a mighty punch.

INFECTION, IMMUNITY, AND IMBALANCE

I mentioned that when you first realize that you have been colonized by microbiota you might be tempted to purge your body of them, but that it would not be a wise thing to do. Yet we all know that some of these species can cause havoc. Some bacteria and viruses, not to mention protozoans, amoebae, and fungi, can even be deadly. Although avoiding contact is your first line of defense, your *strongest* line of defense is the other species of microbiota that populate your gut. As I have already mentioned, the colonies naturally like to do what other life forms do. They like to reproduce, so they compete for space and food. This competition means that some forms of microbiota (in a healthy gut) work to keep other forms in check.

When a few dangerous units of a particular species first get inside your body, they must multiply enough to overcome their natural rivals, and then they must overcome the specialized cells that are generated by your protective immune system. Although it is true that some species are incredibly virulent (no pun intended) most are not that lethal and can be dealt with by the other species. When these other species can't handle matters, then the cells produced by your immune system kick in. But that first line of defense is there only if your gut has rich and diverse colonies.

So rather than focusing on the fear of dangerous agents or on flushing foreign life forms from your body, I prefer to encourage you to maintain healthy and active populations of microbiota that will feed upon the species that can do you harm.

The colonies within your gut, therefore, are in a continuous process of sorting things out amongst themselves, and for the most part need one another. The separate species are busy creating a balance that helps to keep you healthy. If some species lose too much ground and are starving for space and food, the community can easily slide into an unhealthy imbalance. Even if the overly successful species are otherwise benign (they don't have to be lethal ones) an overgrowth can cause problems. To be clear, it is the diversity of the microbiota in your gut that will help you.

Because of the complexity of the makeup of these colonies (hundreds of species are present at any one time) we don't really know what the proper balance is for us humans, much less each person. But a very good way to tell if you are out of balance is that good ol' friend of yours, awareness. If you begin to notice that you react badly to common foods, or are unable to digest food and always feel tired and listless, or if you have to admit that you don't often feel well, then I would say that you are halfway to health. Why halfway? Because you have begun to unwind and to bring an inner awareness to your gut. And you are now being honest about the way you really feel. Later, I'll discuss in more specific terms about how you can tell if you have an imbalance.

IMBALANCE, BIRTH, AND DEVELOPING TOGETHER

I've said that an imbalance in your gut microbiota can be problematic, but before seeing why, let's consider how it could have come about in the first place.

It's a complex story, but I would start by noting that the natural environment is much less diverse than it has been. I think it is indisputable that over the last many decades there has been a significant amount of soil, ocean, and freshwater degradation. With a less diverse environment, we are exposed to a less diverse universe of microscopic living forms. The rich diversity of the past could have included microbes that helped our immunity and overall health, and if so, they've gone missing.

Related to environmental degradation is the way our food is currently grown. One unforeseen cost of industrial-scale farming is that it too alters the diversity of the microbial universe. Modern farming practices, with their emphasis on monoculture, limit our food choices and, because microbes live on and in the food we eat, limit what is available to our gut in the way of microbes.

The quality too of most of the food on offer is much less rich. It's not meeting the nutritive needs of our somatic cells and it seems to be starving our once-healthy gut colonies. Although modern farming has given us a plethora of calories (even if they are unevenly distributed) many of them are empty calories anyway. Empty calories don't do much beyond keep us alive, and they encourage an unhealthy imbalance in our colonies of gut bacteria.

Also, most of us who live in developed countries continue to have less and less contact with the natural environment, and nearly zero participation in the growing, harvesting, and even cooking of our food. It's hard to get a healthy exposure to the microscopic universe when you spend most of your days indoors and as uninvolved as possible with your sustenance. Therefore, I believe that with the equally undeniable progress that comes with civilized life, there has also come a great measure of unhelpful sterilization and a general disassociation with the natural world.

An attendant phenomenon to corporate farming and city life is the problem of the overuse of antibiotics. If you grew up like I did, then you've had plenty of instances where the doctor administered antibiotics, whether warranted or not. Unfortunately, antibiotics are indiscriminate in their killing of the little guys, but also incomplete. Each time you got sick and dutifully took your dosages, your gut had to rebuild from a base composed of the survivors. This was not a situation that brought forth balance. Keep in mind that your childhood exposure to antibiotics also included the ones used in the industrial-scale farming that made meat and fish affordable. These antibiotics did not disappear after they were used to fatten up the animals for market. They ended up somewhere, usually in the water that we all drink. The same was true for the antibiotics in medical practice that were overused for decades and remain widespread. They too ended up in the water supply. (And the problem continues to this day.)

In my practice I encounter many people who have had, like I had, serious medical issues that required hospitalization and the requisite life-saving antibiotic treatments. So I'm not speaking against antibiotics per se, I'm only trying to alert you to the fact that there is a price to be paid, often discovered much later, and that price is having to find a way to rebuild a healthy gut.

The topics of environmental degradation, modern farming, and the overuse of antibiotics are thoroughly discussed and debated elsewhere, and lest I devolve into overtly political rants (I would most likely be preaching to the choir) I will instead focus on things that apply more directly to your health.

Previously, I mentioned that when you were born you were baptized with a generous portion of microbes living in the mucosal, rich slipperiness of the birth canal. Yet many people did not have that right of passage. Instead, some of you joined the world via cesarean birth. The question is, if you had a cesarean birth, did you miss out on a hearty implantation of the vaginal microbiota? Well, the answer is, unfortunately, yes. This type of birth is getting increasingly popular and so the problem is now beginning to be addressed. Some medical professionals are now testing if it is effective to swipe a baby's mouth, face, and skin with a gauze that had been placed in the mother's vagina. Hopefully that will prove to be of benefit, but if you are now an adult who was born cesarean I don't think you will have to do a similar procedure! Later I'll be recommending more pleasant ways to check for and correct any imbalance you might have.

Yet even if you were lucky enough to have a natural birth, it is more likely than not that your mother's microbiota was somewhat out of whack. Environmental and agricultural problems, and antibiotic overuse, have been going on for at least several generations. So your mother might have very well been out of balance and you inherited whatever she had. To be frank, I suspect that many of you had, like me, a mother devoted more to sugar than to actual food. A sugary diet is one of the most significant factors in promoting a gut microbiota imbalance. Anyone who has bounced back from a yeast overgrowth by eating less sugar, fruits, and grains can tell you that.

There is another very important consideration that I'd like to mention. It may seem obvious but I think it bears pointing out. When a child is born, she is not fully developed, especially neurologically. The first three years are key because it is during those first three years that the natural and social environment, *and* the diet of both mother and child, will set up the patterns in the brain *and* in the gut that can persist throughout life. Although it gives me no pleasure to emphasize this fact, it is what it is. But please remember that we all share this environmentally depleted environment and this ramped-up and stressed-out world and, like it or not, we're all going to have to heal together. The good news is that your gut is alive and amenable to therapy, and your brain is a squishy assemblage of changeable genius.

THE MICROBIOME

Knowing that trillions of foreign cells reside in your intestines, and that this is a natural state of affairs that has been going on in your ancestors' guts for eons, and that the hundreds of species that have colonized your gut have evolved together and so will inevitably work out some sort of balance amongst themselves, you might be tempted to think that none of this is a big deal. You might think that, as long as you don't become infected with a dangerous virus or eat food tainted with bad bacteria, you don't need to worry about the microbiota in your gut. Perhaps you might think the little guys are just along for the ride and that it's just a matter of carrying around an extra three pounds that you'd rather not have. Or you might think if you do have an imbalance, you'll only suffer an occasional yeast flare-up or maybe a cold or two during the winter.

Well, I suppose some people are so healthy they can give little thought to this vast number of cells that is part and parcel of themselves. But for the rest of us, we must look at why and how the microbiota can impact our health. Of course the topic is complex and the scientists who are busy studying all the aspects of the microscopic world admit that they have much more to learn. So the details are not yet available, but what is known is important, especially for anyone saddled with ongoing symptoms, a vague diagnosis, unknown solutions for discomfort, or a listless lack of progress. I believe there are two general, overarching concepts that have the potential to change the way you seek to restore your health.

As I have mentioned, the microbiota have coevolved with you, their human host, and so have become an intricate part of your digestive process. In fact, some of your gut microbiota obtain their nutrition from the food you eat while at the same time they aid in the process of breaking down that food. Other species make vitamins, including B^{12}, folic acid, biotin, and vitamin K. The key here is that some species are beneficial in this regard and others may, for example, be too efficient at extracting energy from carbohydrates, and thereby providing too much energy at one time, requiring the body to store the extra energy as fat. Other species depend so much on certain types of food that they could be causing the intermittent or the incessant cravings that might be getting in the way of your dietary ambitions. All this activity creates small molecules (metabolites) and by-products that can get into the blood and affect the other organs such as the stomach, pancreas, and liver, or even your blood vessels, heart, and brain.

Another reason why these little guys are important is that most of these trillions of cells have DNA. The collection of all this genetic material is properly called the microbiome. The expression of these genes can outnumber human genome expression significantly, as much as by a hundred to one. The experts are beginning to tell us that we need to get used to the notion that we humans are in fact a supraorganism, a blend of human and microbe, and that our health outcomes, our psychology, and even our individual personality traits are determined by this blend of genes. That may strike you as more science fiction than science, so here I only want to point out two things: one is that the recent hope for (and the hype surrounding) a revolution in diagnostics and pharmaceutical treatments based on the human genome might have been premature. The other is that some of this genetic material of the microbiome can end up floating around in your body, and it can have an enormous impact on your immune and nervous systems.

THE GUT BRAIN

Whenever one of my clients seems to hit a plateau in the quest for health, more often than not an imbalance in the gut microbiota becomes the prime suspect.

Yet I often wonder how the microbiota and its gene pool, the microbiome, can have such an impact. I wonder because, in a way, these little guys live on what is really an external surface of the body. For they have merely settled into the inner part of the hollow digestive tube, which is, when you think about it, basically a channel running through your body. Through this channel flows the material we call food and beverages, but none of that gets inside of our bodies without first being broken down and carefully monitored before it is assimilated. So how can the rest of the body be subject to the molecular activity and genetic makeup of the microbiota? And how can the seemingly simple, natural, and necessary act of digesting and assimilating food have such an impact on the way we feel?

The answer that I return to, over and over again, is to appreciate the anatomy of the gastrointestinal tube and the nearly miraculous feat of food assimilation. This complex process of assimilation takes place in the very thin folds of the small intestine. (And for some minerals and the recycling of water, in the lining of the colon.) Much of the lining of what I have called the primitive tube, then, is by necessity very thin. It makes for a very delicate frontier between exterior and interior. It is thin and delicate because it must quickly, yet carefully, ferry the molecules from digested food across the border of the lining of the intestine, and into the body.

Remember the three distinct tubes of the embryo that I asked you to envision before? Well, now it's good to think of those three tubes, the digestive, the circulatory, and the nervous system, as having quickly developed and integrated into a team. A fetus receives nutrition via the mother via the umbilicus, but a baby is a full-on being who must eat and digest and assimilate on its own. It accomplishes this by means of the cooperation of these three tubes, which are now fully developed and integrated.

The thin layer of tissue of your digestive tube, the one that separates and protects your internal environment from the external world, needs lots of blood very close to the dividing line. Luckily your circulatory system pervades the digestive tube, bringing blood cells into contact with the cells of the digestive lining so that they can pick up the molecules of digested (broken down) food, and get them transported into the body for sorting and further distribution. Under the conditions we call health (not ideal or perfect, but good enough) the blood shouldn't be seeping out beyond this thin border. The blood must also be vigilant against foreign bodies sneaking in undetected. When this happens, the foreign bodies are quickly attacked, sealed off, and amazingly, their identities are put into your body's memory data bank. The next time agents of a similar type sneak through, there will be a more rapid and effective response.

I'm sharing my very simplified description of the immune response to point out that the action takes place, for the most part, in the blood within your circulatory system. The chemicals that we call poisons, and the biological agents that we call germs, have the potential to enter the blood, trigger a response, and perhaps overwhelm the body. But much of the time this happens because of an imbalance in the microbiota. If the microbial community in your gut, because of an imbalance, produces too many by-products or DNA-loaded proteins, your immune system can easily get confused and run on overdrive. The result is that you can develop allergies or become particularly sensitive—and reactive—to certain foods.

Under these conditions, especially if they persist over a long period of time, lots of unusual things might happen. Sometimes it means that no matter how much a person eats he can't gain weight. For other people with other microbiota profiles, they can digest carbs but have trouble with fats and proteins, or vice-versa. These are just a few scenarios, and your situation will no doubt be unique because your microbiota and any imbalance will be unique to you. For many people, especially those who are frustrated by their weight loss efforts or plagued with symptoms that don't seem to add up to a clear diagnosis, I believe the gut is the place to look for answers.

Unfortunately, beyond allergies and food sensitivities, much worse things can happen. Your immune system can react in such a way as to turn its vigilance toward your somatic cells and begin to attack various tissues of your own body. If this happens, a person can develop any number of auto-immune diseases. Again, I believe treatment for these diseases must at the very least begin with a thorough investigation of the way the gut is digesting and assimilating food, and a careful effort to rebalance the gut microbiota.

And let's not forget the third embryonic tube, the nervous system. It too has developed from the early embryonic state, and it has grown mightily during the first three years of life. By the time you are an adult it has become fully integrated into the whole system. (And perhaps primed for embodiment, joy, and the other goodies of a well-lived life.) This developed nervous system must oversee the conversion of food into molecular energy and the transport of those molecules across the frontier of your gut lining. To properly do this, your nervous system has burrowed to the very limit of that gut lining, right to the borderland, into the mucosa, the inner layer of the digestive tube.

In its sophistication the nervous system formed a specialized branch that independently monitors and modulates the activity of the gut, and it formed this early on, before completing its development in the brain. This specialized branch is made up of millions of enteric nerves, and it has been famously dubbed the Second Brain, and for good reason, because every part of the primitive digestive tube past the esophagus (the stomach, the small intestine, and the colon) has nerve cells that communicate with one another, independent of the brain in the cranium. Of course the brain in your belly doesn't busy itself, like your other brain, with hearing and making images and thoughts and talking and singing. It is far too busy with a more important task, that of providing your other organs and your primary brain with energy to do all those fun things.

Although still underappreciated, this gut-brain is quite extensive and complicated. There are entire books devoted to its discovery and importance, and if you are having unexplained belly problems that don't seem to resolve, I encourage you to read them. Here, I only want to remind you of something that you probably already know. This extensive nervous system communicates with itself, with your heart, your circulatory and hormonal systems, your digestive tube, and with the rest of your body, via the language of molecular chemicals.

While your gut microbiota is doing its things, growing, reproducing, consuming the foods it craves, and interacting with other species in the community of colonies, it is also producing and exchanging chemicals and proteins that signal information to your belly brain. The enteric nervous system is there to monitor and modulate all the activity of digestion and assimilation, so it's going to be aware of, and affected by, what's going on with your gut microbiota too.

Beyond the fact that a gut imbalance can cause you the occasional bellyache, ongoing pain, or disruptive immune system flare-ups, it can have profound consequences for your health, your emotional state, and mental well-being. Any medication you might be on, must be, just like food, digested and assimilated. If your enteric nervous system is either lighted up already, or in some cases, deadened or otherwise unresponsive, it's going to have trouble making use of these medications.

Also, one of the most surprising and possibly important things I learned about the second brain is that, just like the first brain, it uses many different kinds of neurotransmitters, and that most of the body's serotonin, and much of its dopamine, are found in the gut. This is why it will come as no surprise to me when scientists begin to piece together connections between the microbiota and mood, proclivities, or even personality.

Another important feature of the second brain is that, although it can function independently of the first brain, it is nevertheless connected to it. Two cranial nerve pathways connect the first brain to the gut; one sending signals *from* the brain *to* the belly (yes, your stressful thoughts do negatively impact your digestion) and the other sending signals *from* your belly *to* the diaphragm that powers your breath, and *to* your heart and brain. I believe the health and fitness of this latter pathway, the vagus nerve, will one day be key to understanding some very serious diseases. Already, in the present day, it is key to helping with the many forms of trauma that so many of us have suffered. The emotional connections that all of us are naturally predisposed to make, to one degree or another, are impacted by the health and fitness of the pathway of the vagus nerve. Indeed, the physical reality of what some are now calling the social nervous system is a topic dear to my heart, and if I'm lucky or blessed my husband and I will be given the opportunity to write our next book about it.

Therefore, I want to warn you that even though you might have been taught to politely ignore the minor discomforts of bellyaches and digestive issues, if you ignore them for too long, serious problems can crop up. These problems might at first be mistaken as just a matter of the weight gain that comes with aging and having a more sedentary life. But underneath that all-too-natural phenomenon can lurk an imbalance in your gut, an immune system that is beginning to go haywire, and a nervous system that is losing its tone and freezing up. Under these conditions, relaxing, feeling at ease, digesting, assimilating, staying healthy, and being able to relate and express and accept love, is going to get more and more difficult as time goes by.

So we all need the three developed tubes, the three systems, to work together in harmony. We need them integrated and relaxed, free of undue stress, so that they can fully digest and assimilate the nutrients that will keep your organs healthy, and create the energy to lead a vibrant life. Just as the fetus and the newborn child need the right environments to develop in healthy ways, the adult requires a set of skills to create an internal and an external environment in which to breathe, to relax, to heal, and to nurture herself and others.

Below is the short list of symptoms, problems, and diseases that warrant investigation into matters of the gut. Hopefully they don't apply to *your* gut, but if they do, I hope that you commit to learning more, practice the steps you have already encountered in this book, and go forward with the steps that follow.

Appetite and satiety problems

Bloating

Gas

Acne

Psoriasis

Eczema

Thrush, vaginal yeast, other fungal problems such as recurrent athlete's foot

Diarrhea/Constipation

Inflammatory bowel disease

Dental cavities and gum disease

Malnutrition

Asthma

Allergies

Gastric ulcers

Obesity

Diabetes (type II)

Hardening of the arteries

Celiac and other autoimmune diseases such as early onset (type I) diabetes, multiple sclerosis (MS), and Hashimoto's thyroiditis

Autism

TODD'S STORY

As a sixty-year old, I can look back on my life and see the events that led to my decades-long struggle for health. After a happy and energetic childhood, the first serious mishap came in the late 1960s when, as a teenager, I went to a dermatologist searching for help with acne. He put me on what turned out to be a seven-year prescription of tetracycline. No one, least of all the doctor, knew that long-term use of an antibiotic was dangerous because it strips away good bacteria in the gut that's critical in supporting proper digestion and immunity. Or if anyone did know, they certainly didn't tell me.

The next bad turn was probably the most damaging. In the early '80s I began reading about a new "gay cancer," which would eventually come to be known as HIV-AIDS. Because I already felt weak from a compromised immune system, I convinced myself that I had contracted this new and mysterious disease. After all, I had nearly every symptom, among them stomachaches and exhaustion. Because no diagnostic test was then available, I plummeted into a state of chronic fear and stress. I also felt pangs of guilt over the fact that by dying a terrible death I would alienate my family and friends.

I had to wait nearly two years before a test was developed, but fortunately it turned out that I did not have HIV. But it's no secret that chronic stress and depression are bad for one's health. In my case, it lowered my defenses even more, and it was at this time that I developed a strong sensitivity to chemicals. The first whiff of a newly laid carpet or freshly painted room would bring on headaches, weakness, and a horrible taste in my mouth.

I came up with what I thought was an ingenious idea. To protect myself against the fumes, I stopped fully breathing. I thought, "If I don't inhale the chemicals I'll feel better." I wouldn't take a full breath again for the next twenty years!

During this time I saw a string of doctors: traditional, alternative, and some downright crazy. I tried every prescription, supplement, and concoction these folks prescribed, but each one made me sicker than the next.

My immune system took another blow when my partner and I moved into a converted warehouse loft. We hadn't realized that the neighbor downstairs was a mechanic and operated his business right below us. When his window was open, the fumes from toxic chemicals would rise directly into our loft space, and even with our window shut tight we were invaded by the offensive odors. I began to have severe chest and stomach pain. I was clenching my chest and neck muscles and I had headaches. It became difficult to think straight. I remember one evening driving across the Golden Gate Bridge thinking, "I shouldn't even be driving." Eventually we moved out of the loft, but the symptoms continued.

After these long decades of struggle, a friend suggested that I read a book called *Unwinding The Belly* and that I schedule an appointment with the author. My first response was, "Oh, that's not my problem. My digestion is fine. I can pretty much eat whatever I want. Well, except sugar and dairy." Yet at some intuitive level I knew I had to go. It wasn't until I read somewhere that 80 percent of our immune health comes from the gut that I was convinced I should give bellywork a try.

My very first session gave me a new kind of hope. In the room there was an atmosphere of calm and gentle encouragement, and this seemed to transfer into my body. I felt my chronically rock-hard and bloated belly, but with the simple exercises that I began to learn, it relaxed and softened. I especially liked the "Cat's Paws" touch. Slowly but surely I was able to unlock my chest from its perpetual state of rigidity. I learned to breathe three-dimensionally, and began to understand how my digestive system worked, and how I had been holding fear and possibly even the toxicity of the chemicals in the fascia surrounding my organs. I also learned that this fascia communicated with every other part of my body, and this could explain the pain I felt at various points.

Over time, I was guided to sense what really worked for me in terms of diet, supplements, and exercise, and I began to trust myself more while I worked with my medical practitioners.

A few months after first practicing Unwinding, I experienced an intense breakthrough. In the middle of the night, lying in bed, I felt my rib cage unlock. It was as if an iron cast had just unlocked and fell open. My lungs expanded like a balloon, and they could—finally!—fully inflate. My back sank comfortably into the bed. I could feel the mattress for what seemed like the first time.

That was the beginning of my journey to recovery, the recovery I had sought for so many years.

Unwinding has brought real change. Now I begin each morning with deep breathing, but without pushing or forcing my breath. I simply allow the breath to travel to all parts of my body. I feel the expansiveness of me, and I envision my body as being big in the world rather than restrictive and clenched. Throughout the day I enjoy moving my body; taking the time to breathe and expand my rib cage when I do my stretches and while taking the vigorous walks that I do for my daily exercise. I also routinely give myself digestive massages.

Another big learning: I've become aware that my emotions signal every cell in my body, so if I happen to slip into negative thinking it shows up as symptoms in my body. When I begin to worry that my organs are suffering damage from stress or toxic chemicals, and

I begin to feel bad, I focus my thoughts on being healthy, and any untoward symptoms subside. I believe that *where* I place my focus is *what* I'm likely to get. If I think about the pain in my neck or head, I end up with long-lasting headaches, but if I bring a big, beautiful breath to every part of me, I feel more alive, I get a sense of excitement and anticipation about life, and the headache goes away.

As I began to feel better, I was motivated to explore deeper into the causes of poor health. It's as if I were peeling the proverbial onion. My diet was next up, and I began to change it dramatically. I now see food as an ongoing, daily component of my recovery. I now focus on protein and vegetables, and never eat more in one meal than the size of a fist. This habit has helped my energy level to soar. What I find interesting is all the new changes were inspired by a session with someone who gave me the space to breathe.

Back when I was searching for cures I had seen an acupuncturist on and off. This was just before I began Unwinding. After years of not seeing this acupuncturist, I returned for a follow-up visit. After he did a pulse reading he exclaimed, "Wow! What happened? You're a different person. Your energy is so much stronger. There's spaciousness. You're unblocked and your body is thriving."

I owe my new life to Unwinding. Every day I am grateful, and especially so when I follow through on my new, good habits.

Today my life is so good for me and my partner. Together we run an exciting business that allows us to travel the world. I'm now a grandfather to a two-year old boy who calls me "Boppi." Believe me, I'm putty in his hands, and with my newfound energy, I look forward to chasing him around for many years to come.

I RECEIVE MASSAGE THERAPY REGULARLY; DO I STILL NEED TO UNWIND?

Because my husband and I are trained in many different modalities of massage, we massage each other on a regular basis. We both love receiving massage, and we understand that our experience is enhanced because we both love giving, too. I say this because I want my readers to know that I appreciate what skillful massage can do, and to point out that it can be an incredible resource for couples.

However, we don't want to let a good thing backfire on us. Massage, no matter the type, has its positives, but because it can feel so good and comforting, it might lure us into the mistaken belief that we can passively let healing be done for us, or that healing can magically break out of its own accord. Massage therapy is wonderful for many reasons, but we also want to engage, with sufficient attention and willingness, in self-directed practices that bring us to internal awareness. I think it's best if we do that by means of something simple and direct, so that we can match the practice to what we need at the time.

Unwinding is a specific skill set that opens up what can be an entirely new realm of relaxation and inner body awareness. When a person takes a bit of time out for herself and reconnects with her body and her emotional state, without the distraction of another person or trying to conform to a complicated modality, amazing things happen. This is why I always encourage, and yes, sometimes require, clients that I am seeing on a long-term basis to practice on their own between sessions. Otherwise, the development of self-awareness and the feel of what it is like to travel inside and embody may never arise.

Yes, we need instruction, and perhaps for a time a compassionate and nonjudgmental partner to be there with us. But as with any high-level skill, there comes a time when home practice becomes the heart of the matter. This is the reason why I focus on self-help instruction. To my way of looking at things, without the development of a self-help practice, we are left with depending on an expert or discussing yet another theory. Talking about health is all well and good, but ultimately, health is something that you do; it is an experience. You live it, day in and day out.

Unwinding—and relaxation and embodiment—can at first seem to be mysterious. But much of it is about your nervous system, which is to say it's about learning and understanding yourself in a very tangible way. We touch our skin to sense from the outside what is going on internally, and we breathe to connect from the inside. As we go along, week after week, we are able to feel deeper into our body and to notice the many changes that it goes through in day-to-day life, and year after year.

If we relax and tap into ourselves on a consistent basis we will, over time, fine-tune our awareness. We will know which foods makes us bloat or loads us down, and which foods give us sustained energy. We'll know which activities are right for us and which we'd rather avoid, what makes us upset and stressed, and what makes us content and happy. We'll learn how to self-regulate our stress so that we can deal with just about anyone, and we'll know who we really prefer to be around. We'll know when we are being abused and we'll know who is capable and willing to give and receive our respect and love. And we'll also know when we need to reach out for help or learn something new.

I always remind my students that Unwinding is something different from massage, and this is the reason I will only teach it as a self-help practice. When students want to jump ahead and work on other people, without first embodying and growing in self-awareness, then, for me, they have lost the point. Unfortunately, I am afraid this happens all too often in professional trainings. But when Unwinding is understood as a skill—a tangible form of meditation, if you will—that can open up your body to authentic experience and to live the life you want to live, then we are getting somewhere!

6

Further Steps in Unwinding—
Expanded Lateral Breathing and Digestion

Now that you have explored a bit deeper into your gut and its connection to your body and brain, let's return to sensing into your body. I've introduced a lot of breathing into your life, and I want to continue to do so. Better breathing may be quite a new experience for you, so at this point you will review both Belly and Lateral Breathing. With Expanded Lateral Breathing, you will review what you've learned while at the same time adding a few refinements.

EXPANDED LATERAL BREATHING

With this technique, pay more attention to the subtle ways you may be tightening and straining when trying to draw in air. When you are lying on your back with your legs up, make sure your legs and hips are truly relaxed. Notice if you are tight in the area deep within the pelvis, an area that attaches the thigh to the low back through the hips.

Now try to start the breath a little lower, beginning at a place between the navel and the pelvis. That's the true physical center of the body. It's not on the surface of the belly, but below it, on the inside surface of the spine. That's your center! Really try to feel it opening, receiving the breath first, then from there, expanding out three-dimensionally to fill the whole belly, including the pelvic area, hips, sides, and finally the rib cage.

In the effort to get the breath that low and internal there is one thing to look out for. Check to see that you are not contracting the anal sphincter. You want to relax every muscle and to feel as if the draw of air is bringing the diaphragm down comfortably.

After practicing this more complete Belly Breathing, put it aside temporarily, and again practice the Lateral Breathing exercise (chapter 4) in preparation for the upcoming technique. Loosening up the rib cage will make what you are about to do much easier.

STIMULATING THE DIGESTIVE ORGANS

In this step you are going to be working with many organs that are quite complex. You will be dealing with a lot of tightness and unusual sensations, and stimulating many vital functions within the body. This requires you to repeat the technique many times during a practice session, but only as much as is comfortable. Continue to practice it consistently for many weeks until you feel more comfortable. I am going to keep the description of the technique brief, but understand you will be touching five or six complex organ systems (depending on how you count them). Take your time and work thoroughly.

Starting on the left side, place your left hand on the left rib cage, and use all four fingers of the right hand to massage the area just below the ribs just left of the center. First work the area for a while, feeling if it is tight or painful and evaluating the quality and texture of the skin. Move your hand all along from the bottom of the breastbone down to the last small rib on the side. This may strike you as the same area where you worked the colon, but you are going deeper with your touch. You have already softened this area; now your sensory perception, your intention, your feeling, is penetrating further in. The colon has relaxed, cleared, or even shifted out of the way, if not physically, then energetically. Now you are working the digestive organs of the stomach, spleen, and pancreas.

Next, the technique gets a bit complicated, but once you work through it a few times, following the directions closely, it will soon make sense. (There are also audio and video options available on my website, allisonpost.com.)

Keep the working hand inserted underneath the ribs and as you breathe in again, with the working hand feel the ribs expand, perhaps this time a bit more. As you breathe out, feel the ribs relax toward the center. Repeat this several times. All you are doing here is increasing the overall flexibility of the ribs, just by breathing and contacting them through touch.

Next, without pressing the ribs, use a scooping motion with the fingers to coax the tissue toward the navel.

Repeat this as many times as necessary to feel that the ribs have more relaxed play. The underlying tissue will soften and realign down toward the navel. You can also work the surface of the belly all the way down to the top left of the navel rim. After doing this you should feel as if you can breathe much more easily: your ribs and breastbone are not jutting up and out to the front, and you can really give a good exhale and drop your chest. Of course this may take many months of practice, but you are making major changes to your entire body structure, so there is no rush.

Repeat this technique on the right side. First use the fingers of the left hand to massage firmly but gently the area just below the sternum, down to the lowest rib on the right side. Note the quality of the skin. How does it feel: Is it tight, hard as a rock? Is it hot? Is it electric?

After you have softened it somewhat, repeat the rib cage expansion technique that you have just learned for the left side. After a big exhale, sneak the fingers in firmly under the ribs on the right, then feel further lateral movement on the next inhale. Keep the fingers planted firmly underneath during the exhales, while gently holding the ribs with the other hand. After many repetitions, massage and scoop the tissue down and toward the navel several times.

Keep in mind that you are contacting and clearing the liver and gallbladder, so please do it with compassionate touch and wise intention. You are not trying to bruise yourself. Of course, there are many different kinds of tissue between your fingers and the actual organs but this is how you access the liver and gallbladder. You do it from the inside with breath, from the outside with touch.

Notice any patterns of tension from the periphery to the center or elsewhere. Notice if your back, shoulders, or joints become tired or sore, or feel strange quirks of energy. Please remember that the body heals itself in an unspoken language, so you are not required to come up with logical explanations for these sensations. It isn't necessary, or even useful. If any unexplained emotions arise, that's okay, too—just go ahead and feel them and let them be. There's no better time to do so than when you are alone, relaxed, and being compassionate with yourself. Better now than when you're driving down the freeway, don't you think?

Understanding the Digestive Organs

The vital organs of digestion (and immunity) live under each side of the rib cage (figs. 6.1 and 6.2). In a strict anatomical sense you cannot palpate these organs directly, since they are for the most part deep within the body and tucked up underneath the protective structures of both the ribs and diaphragm. But you are definitely contacting them through the breath and by the internal massage-like movement of the diaphragm. You are also stimulating these organs because you are touching with the intention of transmitting compassionate energy.

With this technique, you are encouraging the delivery of oxygen-rich blood to these organs and you are expanding the space where they live. You are giving them more breathing room and fresher air to breathe. Any waste, tension, or emotional charge can be carried off, making room for supportive nutrients to be carried in by the new, fresh blood. The enhanced exchange of blood stimulates digestive and immune functions within your body.

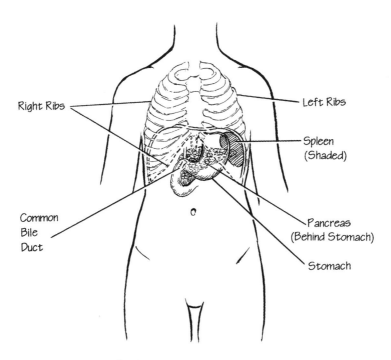

Right Ribs

Left Ribs

Spleen
(Shaded)

Common
Bile
Duct

Pancreas
(Behind Stomach)

Stomach

6.1. Digestive organs—left side.

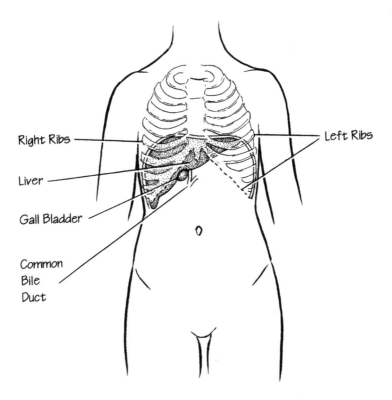

Right Ribs

Liver

Gall Bladder

Common
Bile
Duct

Left Ribs

6.2. Digestive organs—right side.

In chapter 3, you stimulated the flow of lymph tissue in the belly and then worked with the deep abdominal lymph nodes. By working under the left rib cage you are now contacting the largest lymph node of the body, which can be described as the central point of the body's sewer system. This is the spleen. It is basically one large filtering station that cleanses the blood of decaying cellular matter. It also produces the specialized immune cells that stream about the body in the blood. These cells seek out and destroy microorganisms that enter the body from the outside environment.

Now, I know it may be confusing to include the spleen and its immune function in a discussion of digestion. But the blood must be clear and not in a state of hypervigilance in order for the body to properly digest. If you are constantly in a mild, or not so mild, state of immune response, you can't possibly expect to optimally assimilate food energy. Good digestion is a secondary but no less vital benefit of a well-functioning spleen. If your lymph is overloaded by a backlog of body sludge (and remember that the only way to clear the lymph is with deep breathing and lots of movement), you are going to feel sluggish and will not assimilate food properly. And if you are not replenishing the blood with a new crop of immune cells, you won't feel like exercising or breathing or doing much of anything. Immunity and digestion go hand in hand, and impaired function in either creates a vicious cycle that's difficult to break.

While practicing this technique, you may have encountered a particularly lively, uncomfortable place below the breastbone, or just off-center. This is the energy of the gallbladder and the common bile duct. The common bile duct mixes the digestive bile of the liver (stored in the gallbladder) with the digestive enzymes produced by the pancreas. Many people are very sensitive in this area, for good reason. Unfortunately, both the amount and combination of less-than-optimal food unduly taxes the system, and this is one place where indigestion shows up with a vengeance.

When you worked under the center and to the left side of the ribs you softened and calmed the stomach, which is tucked up under the left rib cage. It too is easily disturbed by bad food. The stomach produces the acid that initiates the breakdown of food. That process runs afoul when it is overloaded by quickly consumed large amounts of improper and poorly prepared foods. You will definitely know when this happens because acid reflux is not pleasant, and you may feel the temptation to ignore it by ingesting an antacid formula. But the truth? We need acid to break down food! So the prolonged habit of relying on antacid remedies for temporarily relief is not a solution. It can actually deepen the underlying problem, low stomach acid. There are much better ways to find relief, and you will find what they are by researching—with the support of a good practitioner, perhaps—why you have low stomach acid.

The liver occupies most of the center and upper right side of the belly. It is the underrated and often neglected powerhouse of the body, for it samples and analyzes every food element that is ingested. It stores vitamins, minerals, and food energy from carbohydrate metabolism (glycogen). The liver later distributes this energy to where it needs to go. But if there isn't sufficient muscle mass to help store this energy it ends up converting it into fat. The liver also stores blood for emergency use and regulates the flow of menses, and synthesizes plasma proteins and blood-clotting factors. The liver regulates cholesterol and hormone production, and makes the bile that eventually passes through the gallbladder to help digestion and balance stomach acid.

These are just a few of the liver's functions. Rather than list them all, I will point out that indigestible and otherwise toxic elements, including heavy metals present in drinking water and the residue of medications, are sorted and stored in the liver until it has enough energy to expel them. Indeed, anything that is harmful or toxic to the body is stored in the liver until it has both the opportunity and energy to eliminate it.

The opportunity and energy comes from rest, exercise, relaxation, deep breathing, and eating well. If those things don't happen often enough, the toxic elements end up being passed into the lymph system or stored in fat tissue. The overall result is that the other organs are burdened and the entire body becomes sluggish and tires easily. Anyone suffering from allergies or respiratory problems, whether from food or airborne agents (including air pollution), will also fare better with a clear, healthy, stimulated liver.

The very least you can do for the liver, then, is to give it some positive reinforcement through breath and touch. An atrophied, weakened diaphragm that covers a burdened liver won't signal to you when something is wrong. You must enliven the nerves within the diaphragm and liver. Your liver can't possibly continue to do its countless jobs efficiently when it is cramped within a bound rib cage and starved for fresh, oxygenated blood, so it's vital that you give it compassionate space, touch, and awareness.

The pancreas, on the left side, behind the stomach, produces digestive enzymes. It is quite common for inactive and improperly nourished people to lose the ability to create some of these enzymes. Another vital function of the pancreas is the production of the hormone insulin. Insulin allows the sugar in the blood to be absorbed by the cells. Without proper insulin function, the cells remain unnourished and the body literally starves to death. This is my very basic description of diabetes, and I'm not going to go into any detail here, because we now know that the prevention of adult-onset diabetes is a matter of proper diet, proactive movement, *and* a balanced microbial environment in the gut, *and* effective stress reduction. In fact, a holistic approach is preferable to prevent or work with diabetes or any other disease, and Unwinding will make you feel like taking an active, intelligent interest in that approach.

Working the pancreas and all the digestive organs will help you become more aware of how the organs are doing. You can develop an internal sense of precisely how much to eat, which foods to eat, and when to eat. You will know which foods give you good energy, and which foods bloat you and require more energy than it is worth to digest them.

You will also know when you are zapping yourself with an overkill of sugar. You certainly don't have to be officially diagnosed with diabetes in order to be destabilized and ultimately controlled by sugar highs and lows. Sugar is the most common food element in the American diet, even though it's sometimes hidden. It is something we all have to carefully monitor. My experience and what I've seen with my clients convinces me that we all need to deal with this problem. Sugar has been fed to us from infancy on and most people have yet to experience a meal without it, even though sugar is *not* good for us. In fact, our craving for sugar is most likely driven by an overgrowth of the species of gut bacteria that it thrives on, and consuming more of it will only feed those species, further skewing an unhealthy imbalance of gut microbiota.

The digestive and immune organs are doing the best they can to react to whatever is introduced into the body. Your job is to stay in touch with those reactions and to modify your diet and activity levels accordingly. When you are grounded and centered in your body, at mealtimes you will have the inner strength to say: "Thank you, I've had enough."

SUPERMARKETS AND BEING MINDFUL

Unfortunately, not many people know how to stay in touch with their bodies to the extent of naturally responding to the inner messages, and have difficulty approaching their health in a holistic or preventative manner.

Yet it is no wonder, because every time I have occasion to go into a mainstream supermarket, which is rare, I am shocked to see the sheer volume of products that are devoted to relief of problems caused by improper eating. It seems the more processed, refined, cooked, or packaged products there are, the more remedies appear to counteract their ill-effects. I wander about, trying to find wholesome food among the shelves of pseudo-food. Instead, I encounter more and more aisles devoted to pills and formulas. The inside of the supermarket feels more like a hospital dispensary than a market. There are antacids, constipation and diarrhea formulas, pills for headaches, and painkillers for every part of the body, antihistamines, antifungal ointments, anti-reflux pills, and so on.

Sure, we all have emergencies once in awhile, but when the remedy aisles take up more space than the truly edible food section, there's something amiss.

What are all these products anyway? If the food at the supermarkets were really wholesome, we wouldn't need so many remedies. Basically, all these "anti-this and anti-thats" (as I call them) are meant to allow you to ignore the discomfort of the natural, healthy reactions of the body to bad food. Their job is to suppress symptoms. However, symptoms are simply signs. Symptoms do you the favor of trying to tell you that something within the body is not right, that digestion is not happening in the proper manner. The more you suppress symptoms, ignoring and hiding the problems, the more the body weakens. It may take years to manifest, but disease will be the end result of depending on these products and failing to deal with internal imbalances.

Of course, there is not a one-to-one correlation between disease and products used to disguise the ill-effects of bad food, because that's not the way disease works. It is not a question of which foods or pills cause illness. The cause of most of our physical problems is ignorance and continued unwillingness to listen to the body. The question is: Do you want to continue resorting to symptom-suppressants until you graduate to the pharmacy (also now at the supermarket)?

I know there are a few very serious and horribly painful diseases whose causes are not really understood by scientists, which make them all the more frightening. In essence, the medical system is meant to treat those terrible diseases along with various infectious agents and wounds. But, unfortunately, we live in a consumerist world, and this can negatively influence our approach to health. Advertisers attempt to convince you that personal health is just a matter of buying the right brand of remedy, and that getting well is as easy, quick, and convenient as popping dinner into the microwave. That the commercial aspect of medicine is relentlessly marketed to you does not mean you have to remain uninvolved and passive in the relationship with your body.

I believe that eating natural, whole, unprocessed foods—along with engagement with activities that add strength and endurance and fun to your life—is the true remedy. And I believe that a reliance on an overabundance of supplements or a dependency on pharmaceuticals only gets in the way. Breathing, moving in the way that will get you fit, and finding what serves you in your daily life is key.

Therefore, the step I'd like for you to take here is one of focus, simple but direct awareness. Every time you are about to enter a supermarket, consider doing the following. First, in the parking lot, take a little time before going in and consider the fact that it's not just another store. A market is where you are trading your time and labor, in the form of money, for nutritive sustenance, the very essence of your physical life. I call this mini-technique *feel the wheel*. It's just a matter of taking a breath while you gently hold the steering wheel in your car (or maybe the handlebars on your bike) and realizing that you're not here because you are literally starving, and you're not here for entertainment. You are setting yourself up to make a positive impact upon your health. Second, when you are in the store and encounter the remedy aisle (hopefully by making a wrong turn) you remember what I've said here. Before you reach for a remedy, pause to ask yourself if you're not putting off what you really want for yet another day. Third, remember that you might very well have better choices, such as the farmers market, a health-food store, or a local shop that caters to your needs.

I sincerely say to you that there is nothing quite like finding out what you really want to eat and what you really want out of life. It's done by feeling the state of your digestion, sensing your heartbeat, and by relaxing into a better, more balanced state of mind and of health.

LISA'S STORY

When I had my first Unwinding I was suffering from diarrhea and constipation, bleeding hemorrhoids, and a bleeding, infected fissure in my rectum. I was in tremendous pain. I was doing everything that my nutritionist and rectal surgeon were telling me to do in order to heal my digestive tract and hopefully heal the fissure. I was taking Pepto-Bismol, Jarodophilus, Citrucil, NutriJoint, ginger, goldenseal, rutin, and peppermint tea. I was also soaking the fissure in Vitamin C, applying Vitamin A, and using a salve. But I was still bleeding. I could not have a bowel movement without first soaking in a bath and then applying glyceryl trinitrate ointment to numb the area around the fissure. Even so, it was incredibly painful and I would cry each time. The rectal surgeon suggested surgery to cut out the fissure and surrounding infected area. I was hesitant because I would be missing work for three weeks, but I felt that I had no choice. I did not see the bigger picture.

A massage therapist I was seeing at the time recommended that I make an appointment to learn Unwinding. Before the first session I made a record of my diet. I still have it. Each day was the same. I ate a can of tuna for my protein, combined with pretzels, prunes, and butterscotch candy. I ate the same thing every day! Tuna was my only source of protein, and I had no vegetables in my diet whatsoever. My nutritionist strongly believed in supplements, so in addition to the above remedies, she also had me taking a multivitamin, magnesium, calcium, cod liver oil, vitamin C, silica, and kelp. I also took vitamins for my hair, skin, and nails. But obviously, these did not make up for my poor diet.

During my Unwinding session I realized that I should talk to my nutritionist about removing wheat, dairy and, if possible, sugar from my diet. (Didn't wheat and dairy make up virtually every possible food?) And moreover, I had to admit that I was addicted to pretzels. But I learned about wheat-free breads, such as kamut and spelt, and I was introduced to corn and rice pasta. Also, I learned that I could eat something different every day (a revelation to me), and that I could be eating vegetables like kale, broccoli, and arugula.

After the session I went to the local organic health food store for the first time in my life. Looking back on that first visit, I remember how foreign and scary all of that multicolored food seemed to me. But today, the supermarket chain store seems unusual. My health food store and the local farmers market are places with a special feeling because there's a connection between what they provide and who I am.

It was very hard at first to start this new diet, where I would eat something different every day: a different vegetable, a different protein, and a different fruit. I kept a journal of my meals at first, every day. After only two days on my new diet I experienced interesting changes. I quote my journal: "the most formed stools I have had in a long time." Then I wrote in my journal that I was no longer bleeding and no longer in pain.

I went back to the rectal surgeon about a week after I had started my new diet, and he discovered that the fissure had completely healed. I am still wheat-free, dairy-free, and sugar-free, though I never thought I would be able to do it. I am so happy that I don't have to live with pain and blood every day. Once in a while I will have a hemorrhoidal flare-up, but it is minor and it is typically when I have become somewhat lazy about eating vegetables. Becoming more conscious of my diet again makes the hemorrhoids go away.

Additionally, I learned how to breathe. I didn't realize that I incessantly held my breath until I started to unwind. Growing up in an abusive home, I had learned to hold my breath in fear. I somehow managed to succeed as an adult, but at the age of twenty-nine I was still basically holding my breath. Moreover, when I did breathe, it was a very shallow breath that reached down only so far as my chest and no further than that. It's still an ongoing challenge—I haven't completely overcome this problem—but I continue to practice. Remembering to breathe fully even five times a day is still five times more than before.

With learning how to breathe came the lesson of learning to live in my body. Taking care of my body through eating healthy, natural foods, I began to really feel what I was putting into it. Before, I knew that I was bleeding through the rectum, but I did not relate what I was eating and how I was breathing to what was happening in my rectal area. I know that it sounds unbelievable that I could go through my life so unconscious of my body, but I did. I didn't see the connections between all the different aspects of my life and I had compartmentalized my diet, my job, and my breathing—and my bleeding.

One of the most important things that I've learned is to depend on myself. I had become accustomed to practitioners who either rushed me out of the door, or ones who made me feel like I couldn't make it through life without their various products and supplements. The practice of Unwinding has taught me how to take care of myself by listening to what my body tells me.

Through all of these lessons, I became conscious of what I was doing. I was in a job that was contributing to an unhealthy lifestyle. I was not healthy. But it had been the only job I had known since graduating from college. There was safety there, albeit an unhealthy safety. I had felt too sickly and scared to leave. As I started to get better I was able to visualize what I wanted to do with my life. I quit my job and went back to school to get my doctorate in psychology. I now live a life where I can focus on the healthy me, not the sick me. And I can serve others, with health and happiness as my focus. Unwinding has been like a nurturing teacher, bringing me to what I thought were impossible places, with a guiding hand that is loving and gentle. I have changed so much, and yet this feels like just the beginning.

CAN YOU BE MORE SPECIFIC ABOUT WHAT YOU MEAN BY A PROPER DIET?

It is my fervent wish that more and more people give up their obsession with weight loss and fad diets and instead develop a taste for fresh fruits and a wide variety of vegetables of all colors. I wish more people would drink fresh water as their main beverage. And I wish others would choose not to eat heavily processed, or otherwise nutritionally empty, sugar-laden grains and other products. If people choose to eat meat or dairy, ideally these would be hormone- and antibiotic-free, free-range, and grass-fed. If people did this, they would be consulting doctors for the reason doctors are really needed in the world, and all their activities, studies, and relationships could be conducted in a lighthearted, enjoyable, smooth manner.

Beyond those basic wishes, I am not willing to tell people what they should do. Eating is a very intimate act; at the same time it is a central expression of a culture. The modern American way of growing, packaging, preparing, and eating food reflects the way we do almost everything else. It's not a pretty picture, but it would be futile to try to change it by getting caught up in endless debates about the merits of various diets.

I am asked all the time to recommend a dietary program. However, I rarely walk this path. What I do is work with the clients who are willing to participate in a proactive way, on many levels of healing. But I don't design programs for others. I try to bring people to the point of developing their own programs, prompted by inner acceptance and awareness, not by outward standards and models. If necessary I refer out to practitioners who study the role of gut microbiota and the impact it can have on hormonal and immune function. Ideally, they will value your intuition and understand that stress reduction, deep relaxation, and embodiment go hand in hand with nutrition therapy.

What and how a person eats goes deep into her cells and her soul. It has to do with her relationship to mother and family, her personal history of habits, her genetics, the genetic makeup of her individual microbiome, as well as the current health of her hormonal system. That is why making dietary changes is so difficult. People are often exasperated with the complexity of nutrition and can be tempted to ignore its importance. And yes, addictions, food cravings, and weight issues (and the problems they cause) are real, complicated, and vexing. But that's exactly why I do not advocate one particular diet or lose myself in nutritional minutiae. I can only calmly say that what you eat is vitally important but that you must do the work of finding out what is good for you. I don't believe there is any one right way for everybody. Each person has her own unique mix of factors, so there is no one right way. What's important is to slow down, look at, and feel the consequences of the food you eat.

People currently find themselves in a tough dilemma because they know our way of life is not the best, but they don't know how to slow down enough to do things better. Almost everyone is rushing about without quite knowing why, and feeling guilty about it too. When do they have time to learn the art of eating and living that we admire so much in the Italians and French? How do you find the middle path, the famous "moderation in everything," and manage everything else? Well, that's what is so empowering about relaxing and settling into the natural health of your gut. If you can breathe, detoxify, and clear the center, and then feel from the inside, you will know what you want to be doing when it's time to get up and go, and what you really want to eat. It will become glaringly obvious what substances are harming you. You won't need a diet, a program, or a lifestyle designed by someone else, based on who they are rather than who you are.

What do you want, anyway? Can you think back to your child-hood dreams? What did you intend? Do you really need or want so much *stuff* in your life? Do you really need to be so busy? When you recapture your breath and your *self* within your body, you will know the answers to those questions. I find that the spark at the serene place between exhale and inhale prompts me to love and be loved. But that's just my experience. What's yours?

7

Three-Dimensional Breathing and the Back

For this exercise, you are going to breathe into a place you may have never thought about—the mid and low back.

THREE-DIMENSIONAL BREATHING

On the floor with your knees up, take a moment to become aware of how your back feels now. Feel the mid back and then press the low back into the floor to get a clear sensation of where you are aiming. Then release.

Now, as fully as you can, inhale. Do it as if your belly were a balloon, filling in all directions at once. Pay special attention to the area from behind the navel toward the floor. But try to refrain from flexing any muscles. Breathe slowly and gradually, filling up and feeding the rear portion of the abdomen and then letting the fullness rise to the rib cage. Take in lots of air, lots of relaxation, and take plenty of time.

Repeat until you can feel some movement in the back (fig. 7.1).

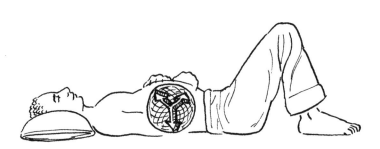

7.1. Three-dimensional breathing. Three-dimensional breathing starts in the center and spreads in all directions. It brings awareness to the whole body.

INTEGRATING THE BACK

Stand up with your feet spread about the width of your hips. Relax your ankles, feet, and toes. Now, slightly bend your knees. Keep the pelvis, chest, and shoulders relaxed. Place your hands on the low back and try the breathing exercise again. Use your hands at the back to offer enough resistance so that you feel the back expanding slightly. There won't be as much play here as with the ribs in Lateral Breathing. The movement is subtle, but you will get the feel for it after you have practiced over a period of time. Eventually you will perceive the breath filling up space from the inside out. It expands from the center of the belly in every direction.

Now check to see if your body is still relaxed, that you haven't stiffened any joints. Shake out your body. Then make loose fists with both hands (fingers together, but soft) and knock on the same place that you held on the low back. (Avoid the spine.) Do this for approximately a full minute, and then rub with the palms or, if you like, the knuckles. You should now feel warm with the blood flowing, but do it only in a comfortable way. You are not giving yourself any bruises, okay? Now your back is awake and happy. No longer is it the lonely and neglected part of the body it once was.

Understanding the Role of the Back

The kidneys reside in the space between the abdominal sac that holds the other organs of the viscera and the mid and low back muscles. The kidneys' main function is to cleanse the blood. They draw out the waste products and deliver them in the form of urine to the bladder to be expelled from the body. The kidneys then empty the clear blood back into the circulatory system. If they failed in their function you would not have long to live, as your body would soon be engulfed in acids.

The kidneys also filter the blood to maintain a balance of minerals in the bloodstream. These minerals must be present in a delicate balance for the heart's electrical function to stay on beat, as it were. Why not thank the kidneys for these absolutely vital functions, and help them out a bit by nourishing them with oxygen that fills your abdomen, sides, back, and front?

Another reason you integrate the back with your belly is to free up your movement. The volition to move emanates from deep within the belly. There is a group of muscles (the psoas) that carry out the impulse to move. The psoas group is important because they run from the mid and low back, pass through the pelvis, and connect to the legs to initiate walking or running. At the mid back, the psoas connects to—you guessed it—that magical breathing muscle, the diaphragm. This particularly auspicious conjunction of muscles is one of the features that make the human body, well, so human-being-like. We don't have fins to swim in water. We don't slither about or crawl on the ground. Nor do we swing among the trees or fly. To move and to do our daily business, we breathe, and we walk, run, dance, or play. It's here, deep within the belly, toward the lower mid back, that the action takes place—movement inspired by the combination of breath and the instincts of the viscera (fig. 7.2).

By contacting this area with relaxed breath, you relate the epicenter of your intention (the belly) with one of the central features of the structure of locomotion (the back). In this way your movement will be free and in accordance with your structure. Stilted, hesitant, jerky, sudden, or forced movements will even out (over time) to a smooth flow that fits your body type. This flow is grounded, in the sense that we humans use gravity and leverage to move. Fluid movement starts in the center. No longer will you be fighting against gravity or defying the laws of physics by thrusting the neck,

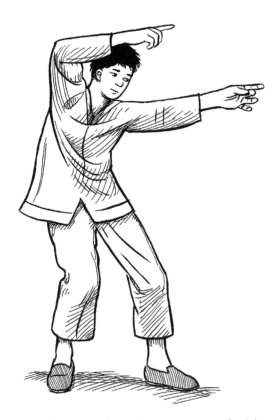

7.2. *Fluid movement.* Movement from the center creates fluid form.

shoulders, or chest to initiate movement. The next time you play sports or move heavy furniture you won't be "throwing your back out" in a thoughtless, breathless moment.

Closely related to the phenomenon of the smooth transfer from breath to movement is the proper function of the adrenal glands. The adrenals are hormonal tissues that sit above both kidneys. The adrenals and the kidneys (two sets of each) are situated in the mid back (fig. 7.3). They sit outside the protective sac of the viscera, so the back muscles are thick and hardy here. (Often the muscles tend to stiffen in an unconscious effort to protect these vital organs.)

The adrenals pump adrenaline and other hormones into the bloodstream to regulate metabolism, blood pressure, and other important bodily functions whenever we are ill or we are reacting to stress. Adrenaline in

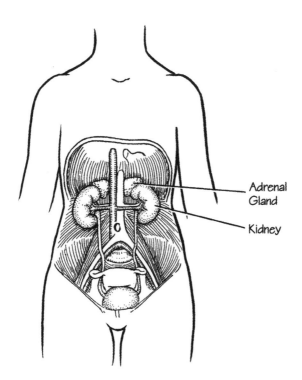

Adrenal
Gland

Kidney

7.3. The kidneys and the adrenal glands.

particular primes the heart and other organs whenever the body is excited or perceives—accurately or mistakenly—that it is in danger. This is the well-known fight or flight response. However, the body can sometimes react differently to illness or stress, and other hormones can create the equally important freeze response.

The problem is that the body doesn't discern which stimuli warrant action and which are false starts. False starts are either by-products of the mind (upsetting memories, worry, fear, or paranoia), incessant, low-grade annoyances, or the inability to shift into a state of relaxation after valid stress. Whether you are being chased by a bear or putting up with that guy talking loudly in the restaurant, stress unconsciously registers in the body in a similar fashion. But usually the body doesn't get to express itself—it doesn't get to either run away or fight—it has to keep on making nice.

As you probably already know, over time these hormonal responses can impede healing from an illness and can be responsible for many common stress-related disorders.

One of the downsides to modern life is that we are generally in a constant state of subconscious excitation and vigilance. Stimulation, even just light and noise, can make us feel alive and vibrant, as if we are in the mix of things and living a full life. Unfortunately, this background atmosphere of excitation can become habit-forming, if not downright addictive. The fact that we have nonstop access to entertainment does not help, and if by chance life does get a bit boring, coffee and other artificial highs can always fill in the gaps. But in my practice I've observed that overwork, keeping too busy, and being attached and attending to electronic devices are the most popular ways to keep those adrenals pumping, leading us to believe that we are really living. For many of my clients, the adrenal glands never get to take the day off, and unfortunately relaxation seems to be unattainable. Also, a burden of responsibility can be too heavy (such as caregiving for a parent) and the effects of past trauma or a disease process can disrupt the relaxation response. As a result, the body can go into a freeze response that we might experience as "overwhelm" or numbing immobilization. Whatever the cause and whichever way the body reacts, the adrenal glands are slowly robbed of their vitality.

It might seem counterintuitive, but when you massage and gently knock on the low back to increase the blood flow in the muscle, you are signaling to the adrenals to take a well-needed vacation. At this stage you will begin to feel how alive and pleasurable relaxation can be. You may even come to prefer relaxation to the ceaseless activity that all too often passes for the full enjoyment of life.

Low back pain is one of the bugaboos of our culture. There is a long-standing, unfortunate tradition of blaming it all on age, the inadequate structure of the spine, and those darn muscles, as if nature's faulty design becomes evident at about the age of forty. Failing to find relief in the various forms of manipulation and surgeries, we blame it on "pinched nerves," without looking into why those nerves, minuscule in themselves, are being so impinged upon. The center of the body, as I've mentioned, is deep within the belly, on the inside surface of the spine. (The spine is very thick in the low back.) It's better to think of the inside edge of the spine as part of the center, and the low back as the backward-facing surface of the belly, because that's exactly what it is. And let's not forget that bloating and inflammation in the intestines, either connected to an imbalance in the gut microbiota and/or adrenal fatigue, can cause low back pain.

As for microscopic tears in the spine, which could have been caused by the stress of chronic overstretching without adequate preparation or breathing (weekend warriors and yoga aficionados, take note) the pain can best be managed, in my opinion, with the very same holistic approach I offer in this book.

By pointing out many of the dynamics of the low back, I hope to have suggested new insights as to how pain "suddenly" comes about. I hope that you are as pleasantly surprised as I was when I found out that proper breathing and awareness through breath taught me to move properly. It also taught me to be adamant about not sitting in chairs for more than is absolutely necessary. Breathing three-dimensionally and integrating the back drove away the low-back-pain boogeyman.

I know it can do the same for you.

PAUL'S STORY

When I think back to the time before I learned how to relax and unwind, and pay attention to my diet, I am amazed at how uncomfortable I was. Almost every morning I woke up stiff and groggy, and at work I struggled to find a way to sit so that my back wouldn't hurt. It is depressing to think about how some members of my family used to sometimes try to convince me that pain was something that I had to learn to live with. They were sure that stiff joints and bad backs were hereditary, and so it was something I would have to accept. There were at least several who had tried surgery for back pain, but had found no relief. It was more alarming to me that they seemed perfectly willing to keep following "doctor's orders" about anti-inflammatories and not overdoing it with exercise. Even while they complained about their negative experiences and their continued pain, they refused to consider any other option. To tell the truth, although I couldn't accept their reasoning, I didn't have any idea what to do about my pain.

Luckily, my wife was determined to help me. She would often ask me to go to yoga class with her. Finally I tried it and went to a series of classes. Some of the other people in the class were able to do things I could never do, and although I didn't let that bother me too much, I did try to stretch as far as I could. (Looking back, I realize I probably ignored the advice of the teacher.) For a few hours after each class I would feel exhilarated, then I would become exhausted and sleep for hours. Upon waking my whole body would be sore. I didn't want my wife to give up on me, but I had trouble staying motivated.

Then one weekend I agreed to accompany my wife to what I thought would be a longer, two-day yoga workshop. Once I arrived I saw that the class was something about bellies. I was skeptical but curious.

From the very first moment this class was different. We didn't launch into a series of poses or stretches. First, there was a discussion about the need for real rest, and how there could be different causes for problems, and each person would have a different solution. This discussion had started being about movement and exercise, but soon veered to how different bodies react differently to food, and why.

After that, we did some gentle exercises. These were so fun to do that it reminded me of when I was a kid and my friends and I would often pretend to be Kung fu masters or ninjas, being able to move around in a flowing, silent, and powerful way.

As we continued the exercises, I felt definite, painful limitations. But I was told not to worry about them or to push through, but to approach them with a curiosity, a sort of "huh, look at that" approach. During another slow-moving exercise that was difficult to do, they recommended that I back off a bit, adjust, and find a different way to "get there." They encouraged me to go around obstacles in a gentle, indirect way. I felt that childlike thrill of discovery and anticipation again. I was hooked.

So after the warm-up exercises I was quite willing to lie down and try the breathing exercises. We were told to do them the same way, no need to power through discomfort, just be patient and listen to your body.

During the rest of the weekend I learned several different ways to work on my abdomen. To be sure, I felt some very uncomfortable places in my body that I had never noticed before, and I knew they wouldn't go away in a day or two. But when I felt how these tight places in my gut lit up my back, hips, and hamstrings, that was my eureka moment. I got the connection. My back pain wasn't a matter of genetics, or even if it was, accepting my fate was not the solution. My back pain was more about the fact that I had never really learned to breathe and that my belly was a stranger to me. Underneath an outer layer of mushiness, it was hard as a rock.

After the workshop, I kept up as well as I could on all the warm-up movements, the breathing, and the belly massage. Over the course of several years I learned which foods made me bloat and realized how they contributed to my stiffness and the back pain.

Now, years later, I am virtually pain-free. I'm proud to say that the warm-up exercises have evolved into a more active exercise program, and I concentrate much more on my diet. Whenever I feel stress building up in my body, I go back to what I learned in the workshop. I work on my belly and I am able to nix the stress before it has a chance to settle in.

The best part is that, even though my wife and I have different diets based upon our different makeup and needs—which makes eating together a challenge at times—we don't get impatient with one another, but just breathe through it. And we joke that it just takes more Kung fu in the kitchen and being a couple of menu ninjas when we dine out.

I HAVE BEEN TOLD TO HOLD IN MY ABDOMINAL MUSCLES WHEN I BREATHE AND MOVE. THIS SOUNDS JUST THE OPPO-SITE OF UNWINDING. I'M CONFUSED. CAN YOU CLARIFY THIS FOR ME?

Like many of my clients, I studied ballet in my youth and Pilates later on in life. I've also been a lifelong, avid exerciser, so I certainly understand the emphasis—and sometimes overemphasis—that is placed on the abs and the core. Over the years I've also encountered, and can appreciate, the practice of reverse breathing that is at times advocated in Qigong, T'ai chi, and martial arts.

Yes, it is true that a healthy posture and dynamic movement depend upon a solid foundation. Yet I believe Unwinding is a perfect complement to core fitness because it encourages the development of that solid foundation. At the same time, Unwinding helps us to widen (lengthen, really) our conception of the core, because for me the core is everything but the arms and the legs, and it runs from the bottom of the spine up to the top of your head. Also, I believe that the true strength of muscle is a matter of tonicity and responsiveness rather than a matter of being solid, or firm, or taut.

When we soften and relax the belly with breathing to establish a gentle communication with touch and an inner awareness, we are relearning a very important aspect of health and kinesiology. Muscle tone is created not only by contracting muscle, but by retaining the ability to relax, sense within, and replenish muscle, fascia, and nervous tissue.

A muscle (or, more realistically, a group of muscles) must also be able to relax for the set of nearby muscles to contract with any grace and force. It is this dynamic that creates fluid movement. I believe anyone versed in exercise, sports, dance, or other forms of enhanced, powerful movement would agree that tight muscles inhibit performance, and a muscle that cannot relax will soon weaken and its associated tendons and ligaments are well on the way to injury.

When we unwind, we are not only talking about the ability to relax muscle. We are invigorating the fascia, nerves, blood and lymph vessels that run through muscles. This is important if we want to retain the brain's connection to the muscles and our perception of movement in the joints. This connection to the nervous system makes for full activation of muscle, a better range of motion, and efficient movement. Blood, oxygen, and nerve responses need free flow throughout the body to carry away waste and to activate muscle. That's not going to happen if we don't combine contraction, relaxation, and rest. This nervous system connection applies to any muscle of the center or core, and this is why I think it is better to be relaxed and embodied if we want to get the most out of our exercise and our movement.

What with all the tension and stress that just being alive entails, our muscles can easily get locked into a constant state of contraction. If we put them under even more tension by attempting the impossible of holding them in constant contraction, in an effort to force an artificial ideal of posture and movement, we can inadvertently train our body and psyche to hold on to unhealthy tension. For a while we might appear to be stronger, younger, thinner, or sexier, but eventually the overall system suffers depletion. A truly strong muscle can relax and contract with natural power when needed. Although some muscle groups remain in longer-term activation over time, to provide protection to the spine and to maintain posture, they must also be able to relax to create gait, agility, and authentic poise while moving.

It's not just about Unwinding, however. Remember that the muscles of the core, no matter how fit they may appear, need to regenerate during sleep. The belly and the entire system must be healed and replenished daily (nightly), on a cellular level and as a whole, so that it can be ready for more movement and expression. And let's not forget a third and vital feature of muscle—that of elasticity or the ability to stretch. A fit, strong muscle can do that too.

Isn't it amazing, the things muscle can do?

Furthermore, when you are in a state of dysbiosis (microbial imbalance or maladaptation), and your gut is bloated due to an inability to digest some foods, or your tissue is inflamed due to an untoward immune response, it will be increasingly difficult for your body to find the energy to keep your core muscles in dynamic, free-flowing response. Indeed, an inability to maintain tonicity in the center (normally and unhelpfully interpreted as being "fat") is a sign that you might need to look into balancing your gut microbiota, regardless of how good your exercise program is. In addition, you might have to suss out if your adrenals are fatigued.

It's incredibly empowering to consider how muscle tissue can do many things, and that it accomplishes it in coordination with the nerves, blood, and fascia—and ultimately with a healthy gut. So please do strengthen your core—your whole core—and use Unwinding to enhance your experience, because it is my wish that you can love your muscles, your abs, and your core because they are potentially just as strong and supple and flexible and multifaceted as *you* can be.

8

Advanced Steps in Unwinding— Connected Breathing, the Inner Voice, and Bone

Your diligent practice has prepared you for the next phase, Connected Breathing. Now you are ready for the full breathing that is the human part of your nature. The body possesses the structure and ability for capacious inspiration and a full life that goes with it. It is the natural legacy that your ancestors have bestowed upon you. You have a right to that legacy, and now you are going to claim it! How? In the same way as with everything in Unwinding: unforced, effortlessly, gracefully.

CONNECTED BREATHING

Start on the floor with your knees up. Breathe a few times into the belly. Then expand that to include Lateral Breathing. Rest a bit. Now start again with Belly and Lateral Breathing together, and after a few repetitions, fill out the back too.

You can put your hands on your belly to make sure you fill up there first, then move your hands to your rib cage, and then feel your back expanding against the floor. Do this several times, the breath expanding out from the center, three-dimensionally, in all directions. Rest again for a few moments. Resume breathing, combining the Belly, Lateral, and Three-Dimensional Breathing steps, filling the entire abdomen up like a balloon. When the abdomen is really full, breathe in even more, letting the chest rise and expand, filling with air, all the way up the ribs to the collarbone. Now the muscles of the ribs and chest are moving (because they are relaxed); the neck, throat, and tongue are relaxed; and the mid and upper lobes of the lungs are given ample room to enrich with oxygen.

As with all the previous breathing instruction, it is very important to remember to inhale through the nose and to exhale through the mouth with the lips and jaw relaxed.

Also, when you exhale, let the upper chest collapse first, then the sides of the ribs, and finally let the belly fall inward (fig. 8.1A). This can take some getting used to. It may take many weeks of practice before you get it. It is a very specific practice, but keep trying. Many people can learn to inhale fully into all areas of the lungs, but few actually exhale fully. In your practice you want to develop the habit of expelling all the old, stale air from the deepest reaches of the lungs.

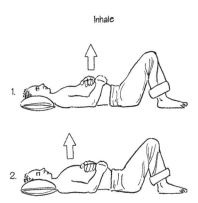

Inhale

8.1A. Connected breathing. First the belly, then the chest.

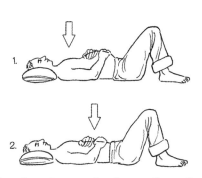

Exhale

8.1B. Connected breathing. Letting the chest collapse first, then the belly.

To better accomplish this, it is helpful to contract the abdominal muscles slightly at the end of the exhale, just to encourage that last bit of air out of the body. After the complete exhale, having tucked the abdominal muscle a bit, wait a moment, relax the muscle, and then let the next inhale arise spontaneously from the center of the belly.

I almost hesitate to pass on this secret, though, if you take it to mean that you now have permission to use the abdominal muscles to do the work of breathing. Please don't throw away all that you have learned. Use this secret as a specific refinement to your technique. Please continue to breathe in the effortless way of Unwinding.

Here are a few more secrets to help you along. After taking oxygen into your entire abdomen, gently swallow before bringing in more oxygen up into the chest. This helps relax the throat. Also, you can employ your hands to guide your breathing from the belly, moving them to your sides and then to your chest, feeling the expansion of each area. Then with your hands, gently encourage the falling of your chest, ribs, and then the belly.

And finally, when you get the hang of Connected Breathing, remember that you have arms, feet, legs, hands, a neck, and head too! Are they relaxed? Are they giving into gravity? Are you aware of the bones that your muscles are attached to? Do the bones feel relaxed and alive? Is blood circulating freely throughout the body?

You would be surprised at some of the things I see in my practice. When a person travels to a state of Connected Breathing, sometimes they first pass through layers of tension that seem to cling to the various tissues of the body. Fingers point straight up, legs shake, feet cramp, arms curl, jaws jut out, brows furrow, hands clench into fists. All of this happens unconsciously, yet it is quite normal. When a person gives total attention to breathing and relaxing the diaphragm and chest, tension springs up elsewhere in the body. This happens because it takes a while for the nervous system to adjust and to reorganize and distribute any tension that is natural and healthy, while shedding any excess.

The point is to feel what is happening to you when you breathe, to be aware of the whole body. Those places where you find yourself stubbornly gripping and cramping right now are the very same places you normally tense up while going about your daily business, and even during sleep. But now you are aware of where and how you hold on to tension. With breathing and awareness you can let the body slip into the change it wants to make, and you can consciously relax. Finally!

After you have mastered all the ways of breathing, including Connected Breathing, it is helpful to practice them while standing. Do it in the same way as you practiced Three-Dimensional Breathing in chapter 7. Spread the feet, relax the knees, and loosen all the joints. Take in air in patient stages. Use the hands to guide the breath into the various places in the suggested order—belly, ribs, back, and chest. Then on the exhale gently encourage the emptying of each area, and slightly tuck in the abdominal muscles at the end of each breath. Pause, and breathe again.

Understanding Connected Breathing

In addition to finding profound, conscious relaxation, connecting the upper body to the belly integrates the physical, emotional, and mental aspects of the entire person. Previously, I said that you do not want your breathing (and life experience) constricted in the shallow, confined spaces of a tense upper body. Likewise, you do not want to merely access the lower instinctual center with Belly Breathing exclusively. You want to marry the two. The heart, lungs, and viscera should function in harmony, all the organ systems working together.

If you have ever known someone suffering from high blood pressure or heart disease, you've seen how the different parts of the body can become disharmonious. The health of the kidneys plays a vital role in those conditions because (as I mentioned in chapter 7) the kidneys and the heart are physiologically interconnected in an amazingly complex way. And that is true of all the organs. The function of the whole body is linked in specific ways by a fascinating chemistry that modern medicine is only just beginning to understand. The heart and lungs may lie above the diaphragm, and the viscera below it, but that does not mean any of the organs operate independent of one another. In an anatomy book, the organs may be neatly defined, identifiable units, and, to put it more crudely, on the dissection table they become easily distinguishable pieces of meat. But chemically (that is, in real life) the body is one vast, intricate, electric, liquid universe. You want to connect the breath (the awareness) to this inner ocean.

THE INNER VOICE

On a different or higher note, within the chest and throat there lives a potential we cannot deny but to our detriment—the voice. The inner voice arises by virtue of *inspire-ation,* and in exhalation it gives expression to our heart's desires. It is vital to reawaken and enliven the chest and throat through relaxation, and to connect them to the intuitive viscera. A spirit cramped within a tight breast that is grasping halfheartedly for air can only repeat what it has been told, report what it has learned is acceptable, and say only what it meekly imagines others want to hear. The true voice speaks for the entire body, the whole person. If it is constrained within the breast or throat it must be literally resuscitated. It will take some doing, though, and much courage.

When I was a child, I was often told that children should be seen and not heard. The older generation held that to be a general rule. That attitude, which is still quite common today, whether overtly or subtly conveyed, quickly leads to the suppression of the natural, buoyant expression of children. And so the story of learning unconsciously to limit breathing continues throughout adolescence (not always the carefree days many adults like to imagine). The stress associated with physical growth and conforming to confusing and restrictive behaviors reflects in patterns of tension within the diaphragm and the entire frame of the body. And so on into adulthood— challenge by challenge, stresses and daily struggles add to the inner tension of the body. A disapproving teacher causes us to react with a restriction in breathing here. A yelling spouse, or sudden shock of a near miss accident, brings more restriction there. On and on it goes, until the body is forced to rely on mere willpower just to go on. We secretly hope that everything will turn out okay in the future. But the future has the nasty habit of always being just around the corner, and the body struggles on, stuck in the rut of stiff habit.

No matter what you have done to manage to survive into adulthood (or no matter how tough the exterior posturing), to some extent fears and tensions have cowered the breath and the free expression of the individual, inner voice. Fear is an unavoidable part of life, and it lives in the structure of your body. Your muscle, fascia, and breathing patterns make up who you are today, which you may find acceptable at times, while at other times you want to feel, do, or be more, better, grander, more complete—living life with more passion and joy than you normally give to it. How is that to be accomplished? Use the full breath to resuscitate the voice. This is why I like to call Connected Breathing "do-it-yourself CPR!"

By the way, when was the last time you felt like singing, or actually did sing, outside in the open? (Or at least outside of the shower?) This is what connected breathing is all about. Well, not only about singing, but also about your voice, the inner voice that wants to rise up and say what it wants to say.

Sometimes in my practice I have the pleasure of witnessing a remarkable event. Clients who initially had come to me with a variety of physical ailments manage, with practice, to connect to their voice. Even though this may present more challenges on the social level (dealing with your family, for example), an interesting phenomenon sometimes takes place. The physical problems melt back into the mysterious void from whence they came.

Therefore, I believe that healing is also a matter of finding a practitioner who can unobtrusively listen to what you have to say while you are making an authentic connection to your voice and integrating it with the instinctual center.

I warn you now that consistently practicing Connected Breathing in a heartfelt way makes it very difficult for you to keep on being unhappy. Your self-expression, opinions, ideas, and creativity can't possibly remain hidden in a tight body, secreted away, behind the places of regret, hurt, anger, and frustration. The more you practice, the less you will need the cigarettes, the alcohol or drugs, the medications, the bad food, the grumpy moods, the blaming, the confusing relationships, to stuff it all down. The inner voice glides upon the breath, conveying the heart's truth. So with the breathing in this book, I bid you take it easy, take it slow, but please do take it! The world is in desperate need of more singers.

INTERCOSTALS

Let's return to technique. First, use the right hand to work the left side. Place the four fingers just below your collarbone and make circular motions, massaging the muscle as you breathe fully into and out of the chest. Work your way from the midline to the shoulder. Continue massaging between each rib, slowly and gently, as you breathe. Now move further down to the lower rib cage, using the same technique. You can use both hands if you like. Massage each rib muscle (the intercostals) and then repeat the procedure on the right side. Feel for any particularly tight spots or areas that feel charged with tension. Don't worry if some places are tight or painful. Almost everyone has a constricted chest and sensitive intercostals (fig. 8.2).

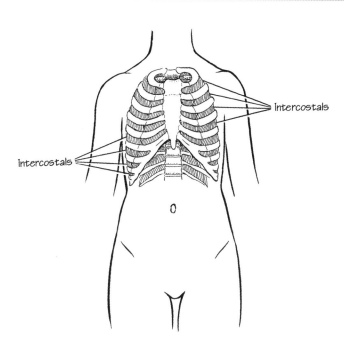

8.2. Intercostals. The ribs and intercostal muscles need expansion and require compassionate touch.

Massage with the intention of acknowledging any electric charge and softening it. Continue to the lower rib cage, where it may feel uncomfortable in a ticklish sort of way. Go ahead and keep breathing and working the ribs, becoming accustomed to the touch. With patience you can overcome these unfamiliar sensations. Pain and any ticklish sensation will soon dissipate, and the touch will quickly become comfortable.

Why You Work the Intercostals

As far as I know, most people have rarely been touched in a healing way on the chest or ribs. As I mentioned in the Connected Breathing exercise, the entire area is constricted and armored against feeling because many of us have shut down our inner voice. A stiff, immobile rib cage and chest inhibit not only the breath but also the movement of the upper body and the pelvis. The arms and legs are restricted in side-to-side and rotational movements by the overly protective shield of tight intercostal muscles. The emotional charge carried in these muscles can be quite severe, resulting in defensive and even hostile reactions to perceived threats. You want to discharge this unnecessary hypervigilance in the upper body, because it limits the movement of the diaphragm and the breathing capacity of the lungs, and can even disrupt the rhythm of the heart. Relaxing the trunk of the body increases its flexibility, allowing more appropriate responses to environmental stress. Previously, I mentioned that lung tissue stores such emotions as unresolved grief, sadness, regret, and the sense of irretrievable loss. Working the intercostals in this manner also helps you to accept and let go of these internal sources of stress.

LOWER ABDOMEN

Bring your attention to your left hip. Place your hands on the belly near the upper surface of the hipbone and "sense in." Begin to work the area with the Cat's Paws technique you learned in chapter 3. Soften the surface and then, on each exhale, touch and sense in a bit deeper. As you work the left-hip area, check to see if there are sensations of heat, cold, or pain. Or perhaps there is a lack of natural sensitivity. One idea is to raise the knee up slightly, feel how the muscle contracts, and then let the knee down. As the muscle relaxes, gently work further in, distinguishing between a contracted abdomen and a relaxed, breath-filled one.

Now transfer to your right hip and repeat, taking your time to massage the area and to sense in.

After you have worked the right side, move to a place in between your two hipbones in the lower center of your belly, below your navel. Breathe deeply and massage gently. Inhale and exhale, while you sense in. If you feel any emotional or physical tension, you can work gently around those areas or take a pause.

When you feel that you have made compassionate contact with your lower abdomen, put your knees down so that your legs are lying relaxed on the floor, bed, or massage table. With your hands on your lower abdomen, take some time to breathe and sense in to this area. Let your hands lightly rest here, your breath rising gently and slowly, your awareness moving all the way down to the bottom of your pelvis, and any remaining tension relaxing on the exhale.

Why You Work the Lower Abdomen

When you first began to unwind you probably discovered that the lower abdomen was very tight, perhaps too tight and too difficult to massage comfortably. With all the breathing and touching you have been practicing, I trust that this area is somewhat softer now.

We've talked about the muscles of forward propulsion, the psoas muscles that attach from the legs to the mid back. The portion of these muscles that is the most difficult to relax is deep within the lower abdomen, just above the hip. Massaging the lower abdomen will relax the psoas and surrounding tissue, allowing them to release any pent-up emotional charge or any protective, and therefore restrictive, pattern of holding. Typically, the psoas muscles have been prompted by the mind to move forward, to charge ahead into life, though possibly not given the complete freedom to physically express those ambitions. The resulting emotional confusion can result in a physical bind at the area of the hipbone. Conscious touch discharges that bound-up, confused energy.

Massaging the lower abdomen also contacts the bladder, another important organ that along with its function of eliminating urine holds the expression of tension within the body, especially the tension of fear. This function, though we all recognize it, goes unheeded. A gentle touch can calmly acknowledge unresolved emotion and smooth out any pattern of constriction held within bladder tissue.

Much of the small intestine resides in the lower abdomen. I have spoken of its vital function often, so I won't repeat it here. But I will reiterate that it is probably in considerable need of nurturing touch, oxygen, and more space for the clear flow of blood so that it can efficiently do its part in digestion.

The lower abdomen also is home to the reproductive, generative organs: the uterus, Fallopian tubes, and in men, the deep yet energetically accessible prostate. These generative organs move the body forward in the same way as the psoas muscles do, but in a different dimension, through the span of generations. They, too, are subject to an overload of toxicity from bad food, emotional tension, inhibited blood and energy circulation, stress, and disharmonious hormonal function.

In my practice I see many women who suffer from bladder infections, fibroids, ovarian cysts, and many men who have problems with inguinal hernias and the prostate gland. Unfortunately, some opt for medication and surgery before seeking alternatives. I believe that quite often these problems can be avoided and effectively relieved with conscious breathing, touch, and the healthy lifestyle that naturally follows from increased awareness.

It seems that the further down the body an area is, the more it is neglected. The lower abdomen is crying out for an oxygen-rich blood flow. There's plenty of oxygen and plenty of blood sloshing around in the upper body. Why not deliver it down to the neglected areas? That way, your journey forward into the world and into the future can be fun again, transforming it from a painful, forced march to a confident, smooth, pleasurable dance.

BONE

I trust that you have proceeded slowly and steadily through all the previous steps, giving yourself plenty of time to absorb the information and to develop new habits of feeling. If that is so, I believe you are undoubtedly much more relaxed and serene than when you started. Your receptivity to valuable internal information has increased, your powers of discernment have improved, and you can now distinguish between real and phantom problems.

It is at this point that we will address bone. You have cleared a lot of tension in the belly, and you have just gingerly approached the thoracic and pelvic girdles (chest and hips). You have also developed an awareness of the spine—the skeletal connection between chest and hips. Now you can apply to the bone the same increased awareness, capacity for feeling, patience, and loving compassion.

If you continue to gently but capaciously breathe and draw your attention to the bone, you will be able to feel an aliveness and vitality that before was, for the most part, outside your consciousness. If you like, you can place one or both hands on a bone that you feel needs nurturing. But you don't have to for this to work. I don't want you to think of this as another thing to do, another technique. It's more of a meditation. If you do touch with your hands, use the gentlest touch you can manage. Primarily, we are touching bone from the inside, with breath.

Usually when we think of bone, too often we picture lifeless material, immovable and hard, much like those model skeletons that you've possibly seen at the doctor's office or in a laboratory classroom at school. But bone is alive, pliable, and ever changing within your body. Blood is produced in some of the bones, and vessels carry blood through the bones just as they carry it anywhere else in the body. Even the marrow is made up of living cells. Bone is permeated with an abundance of nerve tissue. That's why bone is highly sensitive, and it holds a special kind of intelligence, an intelligence waiting for you to put to use.

While in a state of deep, aware relaxation, we can breathe so thoroughly that we can feel oxygenated blood permeate all the bone in the body. In such a state as this, we can travel with our breath and consciousness into our living skeleton, and allow healing to occur there.

At this point of relaxation and feeling, do not be alarmed or afraid of any unusual sensations or what may feel like chaotic electric impulses. This is the bone tissue releasing tension in just the same way that all the tissues in the belly released tension when you touched there. These sensations are bits of information to be processed by the ineffable and unspoken healing wisdom of your body. Try to stay with it, using deep but calm breathing and gentle awareness.

What we are doing by contacting bone in this way is bypassing the place where we usually (with our thinking mind) locate pain—in muscle tissue. That is, we are bypassing muscle tension. We normally register pain in the muscle and tendons, and that's the level where we try to work it away.

However, with conscientious practice you can go around muscle pain, which is mostly just a muscle so used to contracting that it has lost the ability to relax. Now you are so completely relaxed and in a safe healing space that you can either stop protecting with muscle contraction and let go, or you can go ahead and keep contracting, protecting a structure or posture that needs to be there. Or, you may still have pain, a legitimate injury, such as a tear in the muscle and tendon tissue. But now you know much more about this than anyone else could possibly know, and you are properly prepared in body and mind to heal it in an appropriate way.

Muscle contracts as an expression of our intention, conscious or unconscious. Some muscles stay contracted and tight, for all the reasons that we all tend to have different postures, gait, and body language. In a deep feeling state, bypassing muscle tissue, not getting hung up on muscle pain and habitual forms of expression that may or may not be authentic, you are at a place where you can choose to change. You can change to the degree that feels comfortable and fitting at this time. No rush.

It takes trust and lots of courage to go deep; breathing, sinking, traveling deep, letting the muscles and tendons just do what they are doing, and contacting the bone. All this isn't going to happen in a day; it's a skill to develop over time. Keep practicing, and each time be aware that you are expanding your spectrum of feeling. You are training yourself to grasp the sensation of aliveness that exists in a very real, physical way, in the deepest levels of your being. Your chest and hips will free up eventually, and will move and express naturally. And of course, all this feeling can extend to your limbs and cranium too. Your spine, another aspect of your belly and connected to your inner intention, is alive and in constant communication with the rest of you. Now it will loosen up and be an active partner in your dance of life.

So when you are asked why you are doing such and such, or acting in a certain way, you can authentically and truthfully reply: "Because I feel it in my bones!"

CAROL'S STORY

I've always been very independent and proud of the fact that I could be in control of my own body. I had a certain disdain for modern medicine, and chose to give birth to my children at home, which was at that time a very unusual thing to do. Our family used an acupuncturist and a herbalist more often than we consulted our medical doctor. That was until I was thirty-six years old, when things began to change. I started, inexplicably, to experience pain that slowly drained my energy and my sense of independence and personal power.

Over a period of ten years the situation progressively worsened. My periods had always been long and difficult, but I was now beginning to bleed and cramp all month long. I went from using over the counter painkiller pills to prescription drugs. I did everything I knew how to do, but then I lost hope. I broke down and scheduled a hysterectomy. The pain was so constant and severe that I was even looking forward to the operation.

But at the same time I was dreading it. The mere thought of going to the hospital made my body ache in fear. I went to see a massage therapist to calm myself down and she told me about Unwinding. I didn't have any idea of what to expect, but I figured I had nothing to lose.

No one had ever attended to my belly before. In fact, I didn't even let my husband touch my belly. I felt too fat and too vulnerable. At my first Unwinding session I was gently taught to breathe first into the belly, then into the ribs and up into my chest, then to allow the breath to empty at its own uncontrolled pace. With this deep, rhythmic breathing, I began to lightly touch my navel, the area under my ribs, and then down to my pelvic area. At this point the tears began: a huge welling up of sorrow mixed with relief that had no explanation. I felt confused because I could not find words or pictures to make clear what I was experiencing, but I stuck with it. My teacher showed me how to touch the area above my hipbones and toward the center, to my navel. She explained that I was contacting my Fallopian tubes, uterus, and the fibroid tumors that were the source of my physical pain. She also reassured me that it was okay to cry and that it wasn't necessary to explain or make sense of my emotions. She just wanted me to go ahead and feel.

At that moment I realized that no one, including myself, had ever paid attention to or provided comforting care to my womb. Even with all my previous efforts to deal with my problem, I had turned my back on the pain, unwilling and afraid to look at it.

After the session I received written directions on how to do an Unwinding session on myself. I've taken my health back into my own hands. I practiced Unwinding for several days. Soon, the bleeding and the cramping subsided. I canceled the surgery even though my doctor was skeptical and angry. Currently I am having regular periods again, with only a little discomfort on the first day.

I consider the experience a small miracle, a story with a happy ending. The best kind of ending. There was no white knight in shining armor (or a white coat) that came to the rescue. There was only a response to a body that was calling out for the comfort of nurturing touch and the need to be witnessed.

DOES UNWINDING FIT INTO MY STUDY OF YOGA OR SHOULD I ONLY DO ONE OR THE OTHER?

If you are enjoying and finding benefit from it, by all means, continue with yoga. This applies to the study of T'ai chi, Qigong, or any other form of self-cultivation. Unwinding is complementary to them. On the other hand, I've created Unwinding so that it can be used even if you are not currently practicing yoga or Qigong.

We all have to deal with life and want to enjoy it as much as possible. I've designed Unwinding as something anyone can use—people who live, work, and exercise in so-called mainstream ways—but also for those who are exploring the so-called alternative activities. So many people are doing yoga now—and sometimes as their sole fitness activity—that I'm not sure what's mainstream anymore. Most of my clients and students are involved in more than one kind of discipline *and* do something like aerobics *and* meditate, *and* engage in sports. Though they all complain of a lack of time, I think it is wonderful to be alive at this moment in history, isn't it?

More specifically, many of my clients and students are yoga teachers and instructors in meditation. Often, Unwinding comes as a revelation to them, too. That does not mean their disciplines are wrong or they are not doing them correctly; it means there are so many pieces of the puzzle it's difficult to find them all in one place. Unwinding provides one of the key pieces to that puzzle, and so I believe that breathing and self-communication through touch can be done in combination with other practices, but can also be a study in and of itself.

The important thing to keep in mind is that any practice or discipline is most helpful when done with consideration to all the other aspects of preventative and curative health such as breathing, stress reduction, the microbiology of the gut, nutrition, and so much more. We never want to make the mistake of burrowing into one discipline exclusively at the expense of a well-rounded inquiry into health. Unwinding is meant to be a practice of opening up to new and useful information, just as I hope any other form of practice is for you.

Having said that, I know the risk inherent in flitting about between activities or doing too much at once. In the exploration of the art of living there is so much to learn, but it's good to simplify by taking things in small bites. Practice Unwinding and, when the time comes, you will find it all coming together naturally, spontaneously. It's like studying a musical instrument. There's the handling of the instrument, the reading of notation, the comprehension of the various elements, rhythm, and so forth. But then one day, there is music. That's the magic of learning.

9

An Action Plan for Gut Health

In this section we will survey more active steps that you may want to take if you can't seem to break a cycle of discomfort and *dis-ease*. But first I want to warn against skimming through the preliminary steps and deciding to begin your journey here. If you do that, you'd be repeating how many people go about healing, which I believe is missing a key element.

TOWARD A BALANCED LIFE

In chapter 2, I stated what might have seemed just a few years ago a controversial idea; that most therapies and programs, which could be valid in and of themselves, will not work unless you first learn to relax, sense inside your body, and fully inhabit your breath and your center. It bears repeating because in my practice and in my life I've seen so many people, with the best of intentions, fruitlessly cycle through so many programs and protocols in an effort to avoid what is most central to their lives and critical to their very selves.

We all do this, I suppose, especially when we don't feel well and want to get out of pain as soon as possible. I understand. I've done the same. But even if you do find temporary relief or solve a problem here and there, it is inevitable that the same or other symptoms will come along to disrupt the tenuous balance you've managed to find.

Here's why. When discussing the wonderful world of your gut microbiota and microbiome, and how they can have such an impact on your health, I mentioned that many of us were, unfortunately, set up to develop unhealthy patterns from an early age. These patterns developed while the three main systems, the digestive, the nervous, and the circulatory, were integrating in many delicate and subtle ways, from the moment of conception to about the age of three. Given the past and current states of the world and the way we humans go about conceiving and nurturing children, this probably applies to most of us. These patterns create what seems like an unbreakable cycle or feedback loop that continues to create seemingly unrelated problems.

Let's say, for example, that for one reason or another you are subject to lots of stress, and you can't sleep well. Your nervous system never has much of a chance of settling into deep sleep, and so the toxins and decayed proteins from all the creative thinking you did the day before do not drain from the interstitial spaces into the glymphatic network—and onward to your lymphatic vessels in your brain. (Both of these brain structures have been recently discovered). You wake up confused and anxious and proceed without much inspiration. Feeling queasy, you skip breakfast and the exercises you had planned on doing, and later on that day give into foods that your imbalanced microbiota craves. Your digestive system, determined to keep you alive to fight another day, deals with what it's been given while your psyche deals with the guilt. The bellyache that you are just barely aware of (because perhaps you are so accustomed to them) makes it difficult for you to focus and deal with the stress of work.

The cycle continues into another night of restless sleep and suboptimal detoxification. A new day comes, and although you might vary your routine and even force yourself through an exercise routine and a good meal, it's stressful anyway because you have to push yourself to get through the routine and the rest of the day.

As you go along, this cycle might change in scale or appearance, but it really hasn't been disrupted. The stress remains in the nervous system. The digestive system, with its attendant microbiota, is still grappling with the challenges of questionable food, and the blood and circulatory system will be transporting ... well, the molecules of an imbalanced life. Yes, these molecules do affect your thinking and your ability to cope with stress. And so the cycle repeats.

A cycle such as this is difficult to break. It's easy for someone else to tell you to just eat right (or less) and exercise more. But as I've said, this cycle might have been set at an early age, when your three main body systems were coming together in such a way as to survive imbalance, stress, or even trauma. So you don't have to listen to the well-meaning but inadequate solutions proffered by those who might know little about the physiology of human development. The only things you really have to listen to are yourself, your intuition, and perhaps to those frequent bellyaches. You can seek ways to create new patterns and new cycles and find true support for your efforts.

Because you can. Because the good news is that your body also has an ingrained potentiality for cellular and tissue regeneration, and your brain is plastic. Cycles of psychological and physiological disharmony can be broken and new patterns of health and well-being can be created.

Often a family member, friend, or acquaintance talks to me at length about their ailments and complaints. This inevitably leads to a breathless venting of frustration, if not exasperation, at their medical doctors and the health care system. Sometimes, *after* I've opened my heart to theirs in an effort to listen fully, I mention the curious fact that has long been known but rarely discussed in the scientific and medical communities. That our worst problems can be mitigated, if not solved, with enough genuine, thoughtful, and co-relational care. By co-relational care, I mean that care you actively engage in, and when you need help, you find people who are just as engaged in life and health as you are.

So let's take action to disrupt the negative feedback loop that has most likely been cycling round and round between your guts, your blood, and your nerves for a very long time.

A NOTE ON THE ACTION PLAN

The steps that follow are pretty straightforward and do not need as much explanation as the breathing, touch, and embodiment that is involved in relaxation and Unwinding. However, they do require a similar approach in that you will need patience, commitment, and the willingness to periodically reassess and adapt.

Considering the complexity of the body and its connection to the mind, the changes you are asking of yourself are not necessarily easy. Although some of the following steps might seem to be one-offs, that is, you might only have to do them once, it is more likely that, over time, you will have to reassess your overall condition and perform them again. Other steps will require that you continue in your effort for several weeks, if not several months, before you see any change. Also, along the way, you might actually feel a bit worse at times, given that your body will be sloughing off pathogenic microbiota. Also, your cardiovascular and nervous systems will be reacting to new stimuli and going through the same kind of growing pains that are involved with a new exercise regimen. These not-so-comfortable adjustments are natural because your three body systems are reintegrating and laying down healthier patterns of interaction. Finally, some of the steps will definitely need to be repeated periodically because you will no doubt be faced with new challenges and opportunities as you go through the stages of life. In other words, as you age, these steps will most likely become features of your healing and your life. You have a choice as to whether you will plod through them passively and begrudgingly, or to embrace them with curiosity and anticipation. It's up to you.

Whatever you choose to do, please remember that the following steps are just as vital as all the breathing and embodiment. Ideally, you will be doing them concurrently. As you relax and unwind, and become intimate with your body and your very self, these more concrete steps that constitute your action plan can become habits that you cheerfully adapt as part of your life going forward.

BLOOD TESTS AND METABOLIC MARKERS

When you go in for your yearly health screening, the nurse will no doubt record your height, weight, and blood pressure, and pass that information on to your doctor. Your doctor then listens to your heart and lungs, and she'll ask that you get some blood work, if you haven't already done so. What is your doctor looking for? Things you are probably very familiar with by now; fasting blood glucose, cholesterol levels and ratios, and triglycerides, among other considerations. Depending on your condition, there might be more to look at, but these three are the most common. Any outlying numbers, whether high or low or out of proportion, can indicate that you have—or are at risk of developing—what has come to be known as metabolic disorder or metabolic syndrome. That's just a fancy way of saying that, along with high blood pressure, your body is having trouble metabolizing some key ingredients found in most food—sugar (carbs) cholesterol, fat, and protein. Remember, your height/weight ratio—or better, your waist-to-hip circumference ratio—is also considered a significant metabolic marker.

So what is the step that I want you to take here? Well, if any red flag happens to pop up on your blood tests, or if you are in the high or low end of what is normal, that's your signal to develop an active interest in what these red flags really mean. Your doctor will no doubt make the obligatory suggestion to bump up the exercise and make changes to your diet, including the need to monitor portion size. She might also gently hint that alcohol should be consumed in moderation. This is all great advice and you've probably heard it all before, just as I have. But this is the point when your breathing and embodiment skills come into play, because any red flags can be depressing, if not downright scary. No one likes to hear words and phrases such as dyslipidemia, obesity, prediabetes, diabetes, coronary heart disease, stroke, cancer, morbidity, and premature death.

But the scary part begins *after* the doctor has helpfully pointed out metabolic syndrome or metabolic disorder. Because soon after the thoughtful yet brief discussion about diet, exercise, and moderation with alcohol, your doctor will very likely proceed—sometimes within minutes—to recommend one or another medication.

You really can't blame your doctor, because despite the myths we tell each other, behind the relationship between you and your doctor some very powerful forces are at play, forces that have made your doctor almost as powerless as you have been made to be.

Now, I am not saying that you should ignore your doctor's recommendations or reject out of hand the use of medication. After all, he or she is your doctor, and I'm *not* your doctor. What I mean to say is that many of these medications can't heal you. They are not even designed to heal you. This might be a crude way of putting it, but they are for the most part designed to alter the chemistry of your body so that your blood tests read better next time! More generally speaking, these medications work on the symptoms, not on your root problem. Also, many of these medications require that you stay on them for the rest of your life, and they may have very inconvenient, if not damaging, side effects.

My point is that receiving a blood test with a red flag or two should not be the first act in a three-act play, wherein act two is the lecture from your doctor, and act three is when you are handed a prescription for meds. (Paying for all this can be seen as a separate and sometimes incomprehensible play, merely for the fact that the script (bill) is written in what seems like Greek, and because, like ancient Greek drama, this play may be accompanied by the dolorous drones of a chorus.)

Rather, I believe the results of a less than stellar blood test can be the beginning of an enlightening and fruitful journey. You could always envision any red flag as a signal to the beginning of an exciting—but of course pleasantly-paced—race to knowledge and health. In other words, a bad blood test can be an opportunity for you to get involved and find out what all these names and numbers mean. Along the way you may even find out that the tests are too limited and you need more refined tests.

This might at first seem like one big and everlasting chore, but once you get going you will find that being a Sherlock is immensely rewarding. Or, if you don't think you can become your own Sherlock, you can hire one and at least come up to speed enough to tag along as Doctor Watson. If your interest is sparked and you stay with it, either as your own detective or a co-detective, you will at the very least find out what the real problems are, and most likely you will find solutions. I say that in all seriousness, because that is what happened for me and what happens for many of my clients who take on their health challenges with an open heart and an inquisitive mind.

The big idea here is *not* that you should ignore the results of your blood test, or disregard your doctor's advice about paying attention to your diet and exercise. Indeed! I agree with your doctor on those two points. Instead, I prefer that you find out more, especially because having high or low cholesterol, a predisposition for diabetes, and many other conditions, can also have a genetic component. If this is the case, you would probably react better to a different solution or diet than is recommended to others. Reputable companies presently exist that can test for genetic predispositions, so this is no longer a guessing game. (See the Resources section at the end of this book.)

So if you do get a blood test result that is outside the normal range, you do not have to panic out of fear or settle for a solution that seems to be designed only to put you at ease, mitigate symptoms, or might be more suitable for someone else. Instead, it can be something that you can quickly turn into a string of positives. Yes, change is difficult. But it's good to recognize that changing things for the better is one of the more interesting and rewarding things in life that you can do. It's certainly better than taking things for granted or becoming dependent upon dicey medications.

SAYING FAREWELL TO SUGAR

If you've been reading this book from beginning to end, you already know how I feel about sugar and how it has invaded just about every nook and cranny of our food supply. I have also stated that I don't normally give dietary advice. But *added* and *excessive use* of sugar is not really a food but a dangerous poison that has both immediate and chronic negative effects. It also ends up to be just as habit forming, in a negative way, as any other behavior or substance that over-zings the reward chemicals in your belly and brain. Therefore, I don't consider it to be dietary advice when I recommend that you do whatever you can to find a way to cut it from your life. Folks, just to be clear: any time sugar is added, it's excessive.

I feel very strongly that if you want to be healthy in longevity, at some point in your journey it will be necessary for you to break your attachment to unnatural consumption of sugar. No, table sugar and all the other too-readily available forms of added sugar is not what made our brains explode in size and intelligence at one point in our evolutionary path. (That honor may very well go to cooking, but that is a different story.) And unless you are running a marathon in real-time or going into diabetic shock, you don't really need that kind of energy boost.

Once you begin to cut added sugar, you might recognize, like others have, that liking it is not a preference or proclivity or a lifestyle choice, but is indeed just a habit of craving verging on an addiction.

I could list hundreds of reasons why sugar poses a threat to your health, and tell you that it is most likely part of what is blocking you from making progress, but I won't because there are so many good books and other sources about the clear dangers of sugar. (I've added a few in the Resources section to get you started.) There is such good science on this topic that I don't feel compelled to debate the issue. I really do suspect that anyone attempting to rationalize sugar either works for the industry or has become disillusioned by the confusion spread by others who say added sugar in moderation is equivalent to any other form of carbohydrate consumption.

Whenever I have argued about sugar with another person, I realize we are not really discussing the evidence but dealing with the same sort of rigidity, anger, disappointment, and regret that comes with exploring emotional states such as attachment and grief. Under these circumstances the best thing I can do is to offer my listening skills. I can do that with compassion because I too had once, in my youth, used sugar as a substitute for all the good things missing in my life.

I will add that sugar, for most people, is so incredibly difficult to say good-bye to because it sets up hormonal and neurotransmitter signals in the body that create the same kind of feedback loop between body and brain as that created by an addictive drug. On top of that, the yeast and possibly some other species of microbiota in your gut *love* sugar, and so, unfortunately, if you crave sugar you are not only craving it for yourself but for many of those little guys that live inside of you and have grown out of control.

Also, I need to remind you that whatever you read about added and excessive intake of sugar applies to processed grains, most fast foods, and many items marketed one way or another as health food. Even many of the products in your local health food store contain enough added sugar to keep you craving it and to prevent you from balancing your gut microbiota.

The good news is that for many people, once they have taken this step, the craving stops within weeks, if not days. They also begin to feel better immediately and find improvement in whatever health issue they are dealing with. That is what happened to me and every client that I've ever worked with who has taken this step, and I know that no matter what symptoms and conditions you may have, saying farewell to sugar will give you a whole new perspective on life and health.

DIGGING DEEPER WITH A COMPREHENSIVE STOOL ANALYSIS

The following is a very important step in your journey to restore your health. I believe digging deeper than a yearly check up with basic blood tests is something that almost everyone who takes an interest in their own healing will be doing in the future. I would encourage you to consider getting a comprehensive stool analysis even if you fall within the normal limits in metabolic markers but you are still bothered by vague or hard to pin down symptoms like sluggishness, frequent changes in your stools, insomnia, or a constellation of seemingly unrelated symptoms.

Unfortunately, many doctors either won't think further testing is necessary, or they will not begin to treat problems that your blood tests might be pointing toward until you have hit numbers that indicate that you have an identifiable condition or disease. Some doctors may be inclined to prescribe medications for relief of bothersome symptoms without finding out why you're having them, specifically. They might suggest over-the-counter remedies or medications either for constipation, irritable bowel syndrome, and acid reflux ... the list and the products used for generalized gut problems is a long one.

However, you'll never really have a chance of solving the problem if you don't know what the cause is, and partaking in this kind of analysis will give you specific understanding of your ability to digest and assimilate the food you eat. Also, a comprehensive stool analysis will check for imbalances in your microbiota and screen for parasites, yeast, and other fungal infections, and problems with fat and protein absorption.

One way to look at this is that you are taking a survey of that all-important gut tube that I mentioned in chapter 5. A stool test will also measure stomach acids, pancreatic juices, and inflammatory markers such as too much mucus in the stool. You will also get some good clues about any problems you're having with your immunity, hormonal function, and nervous system, and you might even find out that a physical problem is causing you stress or, conversely, that your psychological stress is disturbing your gut or affecting the rest of your body.

Other than the cost and the slight inconvenience of actually collecting your stool over a three-day period, the only difficulty that may arise is convincing your doctor or finding one who is sympathetic to your desire to find answers. But do not despair if you are unable to do this because acupuncturists and functional medicine practitioners can order the tests for you. The important thing is to find someone you trust who is versed in gut medicine so that she can competently help you interpret the results. By doing your own research and coupling that with the counsel of a knowledgeable and communicative practitioner, you should be able to arrive at a meaningful way forward.

I feel that the most important consideration in choosing a professional health care advisor, when tooling down into more specific tests, is to find one who not only has good credentials and comes recommended by those you trust, and who can answer your questions, but is one who can really listen to you. It might seem at times that listening is a lost art, but I know from my own experience that there are some extraordinary people out there, and I am confident that if you have the intention and the persistence, your Sherlock will appear.

A FOOD-ELIMINATION PROTOCOL

After you've taken the heroic step of freeing yourself from the chains of sugar, you might find that your body still doesn't feel quite right and your mind isn't as clear as it used to be. Or perhaps you do feel much better in some ways but you are still being bothered by a symptom or two that have become so familiar that they almost seem a part of your life. Or maybe you are struggling with an autoimmune disease or a constellation of problems that mimic one. For each of these scenarios, and for others I cannot describe because I haven't met you personally, I would encourage you to not lose faith and to stay the course with your sugar-free life, but I would also respectfully suggest that you have more digging to do.

Over the years a person's body changes, and stress takes its toll. Recent, significant trauma (or past trauma that has become part of your somatic response system) can have a dramatic impact on your body's functioning. The upshot is that foods that were once nourishing could now be triggering reactions that make you sick. When your body was young and resilient, and life so entrancing, you might not have been bothered with things that didn't really agree with you in the first place. But you don't have the same quantity of hormones coursing through your system that made it possible to ignore discomfort or pain. You can feel that something is wrong, and it could turn into more serious problems, such as lack of sleep, unexplained weight loss or weight gain, leaky gut syndrome, or a plummet in Vitamin D or hormone levels. (If you are young and having problems, it could be that your youthful hormones are out of balance.)

The real problem is not that we don't want to face change so much as it is sometimes very tricky to discern which food, if any, is causing disturbances. That's because, although it could be due to stress or traumatic experiences, the culprit usually isn't at the food level but at the molecular level.

When we go about our busy lives as best we can, and while we naturally consume a wide variety of ingredients, it is very difficult, if not impossible, to identify and keep track of everything. The different kinds of fats, what seems like an endless list of proteins, and the dubious quality of carbohydrates that we consume over the course of weeks and months seem at first too difficult to track. This is especially true when we realize that most whole foods (as opposed to altered or completely man-made creations) are composed of a combination of all three macronutrients (fats, proteins, carbohydrates) and can include other elements such as fiber and minerals, and in varying ratios. It's this variance of ratios that—basically—explains why foods vary in appearance, texture, and taste, and it's the reason that vegetarians, avid meat eaters, and courageous defenders of traditional cuisines can and will find reasonable justification for their particular approach.

But despite the confusion, do not despair, because you have the benefit of thousands of years of human experimentation behind you, and we humans pretty much know which molecules, depending on your genetic background, individual makeup, and life circumstances, might be the culprit. Again, the foods that contain these molecules might have previously been fine or at least didn't slow you down, but at one time or another in your life they began to cause problems. Possibly they have evolved to become a real health issue for you now.

The list of these suspect foods (containing the offending molecules) include the commonly recognized allergens such as eggs, shellfish, and peanuts. But it also includes—and to some of us very frustratingly so—common things that, as I have said, might have once been innocuous or even good for us but now are not—such as milk, wheat and other grains that have gluten, and oils that are used in processed foods: canola, corn, and soy.

The problem, again, is not that you may be allergic or have developed a serious sensitivity to a certain food or a class of foods such as dairy or carbs. The problem lies in your body's reaction to particular ingredients such as lactose, casein, or gluten. Also, the nearly ubiquitous presence of genetically modified organisms (GMOs) in most processed foods (without labeling) also complicates digestive matters.

In this scenario, the step that becomes necessary is to go through a strict yet sensible elimination protocol. I do not call it an elimination diet for the good reason that it isn't a diet. You probably, like almost everyone, have tried many different diets that have been popular over the years and you might have had some success, but again, the issue here is not one of limiting calories or adopting a lifestyle based on limiting or complete avoidance of one or another macronutrient. Although maintaining a healthy weight is a worthy goal, the issue here is to find out which particular molecules are not being digested properly so that they can work their magic in your body, and which molecules are setting off an immune response that have caused the heretofore inexplicable symptoms and that will weaken and eventually damage your body.

The best way to begin is to arm yourself with enough knowledge to learn how to read packaging labels and to navigate the many tricks that corporations use in an attempt to fool you. (We've listed a good website for this in the Resources section.) In addition you may want to have a good dictionary handy so that you can navigate the scientific jargon you come across in your research.

With these two preliminary steps under your belt you are now ready for an elimination protocol that could possibly take up to ninety days. Your daily consumption will at first seem bland and that is because you are trying to arrive at a neutral place before you start adding back in foods that give variety and richness to life. You'll need as much as ninety days so that your body can make the necessary adjustments it needs to make, given how the patterns of digestion and absorption cycle through your body systems. (nervous, hormonal, immune.) Only after the adjustments take place and the patterns change will you be able to properly estimate the effects of not eating a particular substance. By that time you might be feeling so good you might even forget you're on a protocol. If that is not the case, you move on to another suspect.

If conducting a food-elimination protocol by yourself seems confusing or overwhelming, there are plenty of resources to help you. Many of the leading practitioners of functional or integrative medicine have designed programs, and much of the material you need to get started is inexpensive or free on their websites. If you'd like to get started or to do some preliminary reading on what it's all about, check out the listings in the Resources section and take it from there. If you do decide to find help, keep in mind that all elimination protocols are basically self-directed. You will be the one keeping track of what you eat and, especially, of how you feel, so the breathing and the relaxation that you've learned is going to come in handy here.

My favorite part of conducting periodic food-elimination protocols (I have done them many times for myself) is that I realize that a whole new way of looking at diets and medicine has finally come about. It was always true that standardized tests and broad categories were not enough, and that the focus needs to be on the individual, on her makeup, and on the interplay of life's complexities, the importance of the environment, and the quality of relationships she has with others. It gives me hope that things are evolving in a positive direction. I hope that you will embrace this new, wonderful world that is presently coming forth, one in which medicine recognizes that yes, we are all the same but we are also different, that we change through time, and that we now have the opportunity to explore, discover, and choose what we eat and what we do.

MAKING ADJUSTMENTS WHILE KEEPING WITH YOUR CORE PROGRAM

At this point you've probably found at least a few key issues in your gut-body that may very well explain why you don't feel well, and you are motivated to work on them. Perhaps you've made some progress in cutting out the sugar. Perhaps you've found a sympathetic and skilled practitioner that has helped you suss it all out and will develop a therapy protocol *with* you. If so, that's great, but the step to take now, along with any supplements or herbs or remedies, is to make sure that you not only keep involved in the process but are willing to make the necessary adjustments to your core program. That is, it's vital to recognize that along with a treatment program, you are engaging in fundamental changes that will take place over time and that will apply to the way you live your life.

For example, many times an imbalance in the gut microbiota is at the bottom of a health issue, in particular a dearth of beneficial bacteria, and taking probiotics seems like a reasonable solution. But a few qualifications apply to probiotics. The first is that if you are immunocompromised or taking medications that make you less able to fight off infection, you should first consult with your physician. Probiotics are becoming very popular of late but that doesn't mean they are for everyone. If you decide to take them, you don't have to limit yourself to the pill form, but could consider adding in sugar-free yogurt, kefir, or fermented vegetables to your diet. Also, probiotics (and this goes for any supplement) are not a cure-all and cannot replace the need to make the challenging but vital changes that an unhealthy person needs to make, which for the most part are changes in diet and movement and, yes, relationships to self and others.

Unfortunately, in my practice, I've seen that people will grasp at any solution that resembles the ease of modern medical practice, and probiotics and supplements fit that bill. Although I do take probiotics and supplements, I continuously alternate and refine my regimen, based on my current condition. I don't do so indiscriminately or just because a practitioner told me to. I do it only after careful consideration, and I periodically monitor my reaction through blood tests and especially the way I feel. And more important, I don't consider them a replacement for the three cornerstones of my health—truly good food eaten in a relaxed setting, vigorous yet joyful exercise that is appropriate to my age and current condition, and relationships built on the compassionate communication of the love of truth and the truth of love.

That's saying a lot, and yes, it's easier said than done. But if you go about things slowly and steadily and stick to your purpose, nearly anything is possible. I have found that when I have hit upon a new way of dancing with these core aspects of life, they nearly always strike me, in retrospect, as simpler than I had expected. For example, you will be surprised at how a weekend class in preparing fresh and healthy meals can spark a creative burst of restaurant-free, stress-free, and convivial dining at home. A small changeup in the exercise routine and learning new moves will challenge your muscles, interest your brain, and be joyful to do. And when you take a stab at telling the people who are important to you how you feel and what you want to experience, and listen (and watch carefully) to how they respond, clarity abounds and solutions will arise that may pleasantly surprise you.

So the step here that I recommend is to go ahead with a healing protocol based upon what you find in any blood or stool test, but do so in the wider context of your life and your quest. I believe that a judicious use of beneficial bacteria, herbs, supplements, and remedies can be helpful, but they work their magic when in the field of the positive vibrations of your expressed, healthy desires.

DEEPENING YOUR EMBODIMENT PRACTICE

Having said all of the above, the question you might ask is, "Sounds great, but how can I possibly manage all that?"

The answer, at least the one that I have to offer, is simple. Maybe not easy, but simple. Slow down. Rest. Relax. Breathe. When the time is right—and only you can know when that is—you can choose to go deeper than just Unwinding and partake in further exploration of embodiment. I believe that meditation, or focused awareness, is a fundamental health skill and that you can learn it by practicing to settle inside your body and be with your *self*.

Perhaps you are already an experienced meditator and this strikes you as obvious, or maybe the word "embodiment" confounds you and this sounds silly to you now. Either way, meditation is something that I return to each and every day, even just for a minute or two, yet on and off throughout the day. It keeps me in touch with my inner life, and it helps maintain boundaries with others. An embodiment exploration gives me breathing room to be responsive to others and events, instead of reactive. I become aware of the space around me and what it contains, and that supports and provides a unity to my study of the nitty gritty details of health and medicine and to my evaluation of protocols and programs. And so I believe it would be helpful if it could to do the same for you.

Nowadays, there are online workshops and meditation summits, and maybe even apps for your phone, so you are free to explore and choose what resonates with you. There are also local teachers and meditation groups that meet regularly.

During the course of my life I've sampled many traditions of quiet contemplation, just like many of you have. Over time, my practice has shifted (or evolved, depending upon how you look at it) into something that isn't fancy. I slow down, become neutral and spacious. I notice that what is inside of me and around me has unity. Going deeper into relaxed awareness gives me room to let go of discordant sensations. I begin to feel liquid, and light and heavy at the same time. I become expansive yet held within the embrace of what I call both nature and love. My thoughts retreat and rest, and a quiet awareness and presence arise.

But that's just me. The step I would have you take now is to keep in mind, especially when you are grappling with difficult and painful health issues, that you have at hand many opportunities to safely and gently go deeper into your body and discover what it is that you were born to discover.

I've listed a few points of departure for you in the Resources section, and know that I always extend my hand toward those of you who need to check back in with me—and with your gut and your beautiful belly.

IS IT NECESSARY TO STUDY MORE ANATOMY AND PHYSIOLOGY (A&P)?

You don't have to do so while you progress through the steps required to learn Unwinding. Please remember to keep your practice simple.

But once you are on your way, feeling somewhat unwound and relaxed, you may be more and more curious as to what your gut and your body are all about. You will know when that is. Look at it as your body asking you to take an interest in life and in yourself.

It's a lot of fun to investigate life—how growth and transformation happen. I know that's a funny way to put it, but it's just that the normal definition of A&P, the "study of structure and function," can make it seem more like engineering than a life science. So if you do study more I hope that the A&P doesn't sweep you up into too much abstraction. Too many drawings of lifeless cadavers and uninspired descriptions can lead you to believe we are nothing more than just another unit off the assembly line. That is an unwarranted and depressing outcome of so much study.

I try to remember to look beyond the lifeless bones and pieces of meat and take into my mind's eye the whole picture, in living color, and add in the movement, the touch, the sound, the tastes, and the smells, too! That may sound unpleasant, but it keeps study of our bodies alive and fun.

Many of my students in workshops are health professionals from a variety of fields, and once they've been introduced to relaxation and breathing, the pressure to remember all they know and how they have been taught to know it lifts and evaporates. They actually become overjoyed at the prospect of experiencing the body in nonverbal ways. When they relax and unwind, my students get to experience that knowledge in a physical, hands-on way, as a form of energy and movement within their bodies. For me, that is what studying A&P alongside self-healing is all about. You and I are experimenters and explorers, finding where things are, how they feel, and how they work together as one living body and with the environment.

Studying A&P is also a great way to keep up your motivation for exercise and good eating. When you fall off track, pick up your favorite A&P text. That will get you going again! If you ever experienced that kind of motivation when studying A&P when you were younger, and want to revive it, seek out a few of the very best books and videos and refer to them often.

When I study A&P now, I make sure that I ask myself questions along the way, like: "How does this fit into everything else and into the environment? What would change if the model or cadaver suddenly came to life? And more important, "How can I enjoy my body and my life just the way it is, right now, without focusing on problems and disease? How can I accept and enjoy life as it is without fixing it? How can I feel joy and *just be*?

When I look at the illustrations, I try to fill them out in my imagination into three dimensions, and then color in the life force coursing through it. There's no point studying pictures of cadavers without translating the information to a live person—to myself or to those I care about.

As you can see, I use A&P as motivation, an aid to meditation, and a spark to my creative imagination. I know it might sound strange that when studying A&P I'm inspired to feel joy and *just be*. But that's what it comes down to.

For me. But what about you?

When you have unwound, and have exposed the inner critic that tries to make your body march along in step with all the "shoulds" and "supposed-tos" of a life based on artificial models and abstraction, then you can—do what?

Let intuition spontaneously arise and interact with the world in a natural way. Let the inherent intelligence flow, creating organic health. I know it takes a lot of trust, but that's why we take things slowly, healing and building our personal power step-by-step.

When you have unraveled the tension in the tissue to let life dance to its own rhythms and to all the known and unknown biorhythms, and to the waves of energy that create the rhythms, even if these waves seem chaotic at times, you are on your way. You don't need me (or anyone else) to tell you how to structure your life. When you need more information about your gut and more healthful activity, you will seek it out.

During my workshops, questions about A&P usually lead to deeper, more interesting, philosophical questions. And that's good. The questions go on and on, and round and round. Then there arises in the room an almost palpable fear that all our knowledge, ideas, beliefs, and metaphors add up to nothing, that there may be nothing in life to depend on. Right at that moment, before there is a general retreat to all the limiting beliefs we showed up with, I get everyone up to do some yoga flow or a movement Qigong. Or sometimes I have everyone lie down for a meditative embodiment exploration. Or better, we all break for lunch!

I do this because I want students to infuse book knowledge with living, eating, breathing, feeling, movement, and rest; I want to remind them what it feels like to *just be.*

I do the same whenever clients seem to be drowning in a whirl-pool of confusing problems. Even though there is a straightforward diagnosis by a doctor, the standard treatment isn't working. They try an array of modalities, but make no clear progress. They don't know which alternative formula or protocol to try next, or which books to read. After I have, over the course of several sessions, gently pointed in the direction of gut health and the steps presented in the latter half of this book, I encourage them to go back to the simple basics so that the rest of life doesn't pass by unnoticed. When healing becomes a chore or more of an endless research project than a pleasant dance, I can only offer breathing, touch, awareness, a gentle exercise or two, and the same heartfelt, loving encourage-ment that I offer to you: *Just be!*

RESOURCES

A ninety-five minute digital audio recording is available on our website. It guides you through all the breathing and touch techniques found in this book and also includes a bonus embodiment meditation. To find it, please go to: allisonpost.com. Also available is a video recording that includes step-by-step instruction in Unwinding.

We also recommend the following additional resources:

Calais-Germain, Blandine. *Anatomy of Movement.* Seattle: Eastland Press, 1993.

Cook Karlsen, Micaela. *A Plant-Based Life: Your Complete Guide to Great Food, Radiant Health, Boundless Energy, and a Better Body.* New York: Amacom, 2016.

Desikachar, T. K. V. *The Heart of Yoga.* Rochester, Vermont: Inner Traditions International, 1995.

Doidge, Norman. *The Brain That Changes Itself: Stories of Personal Triumph from the Frontiers of Brain Science.* London: Penguin Books, 2007.

Enders, Giulia. *Gut: The Inside Story of Our Body's Most Underrated Organ.* Vancouver/Berkeley: Greystone Books, 2015.

Ewers, Keesha. *Solving the Autoimmune Puzzle: The Woman's Guide to Reclaiming Emotional Freedom and Vibrant Health.* Issaquah, WA: Samadhi Press, 2017.

Foster, Rick and Hicks, Greg. *How We Choose to be Happy: The 9 Choices of Extremely Happy People—Their Secrets, Their Stories.* New York: Tarcher-Perigee, 2004.

Gates, Donna. *The Body Ecology Diet: Recovering Your Health and Rebuilding Your Immunity.* Carlsbad, CA./New York: Hay House; revised edition 2011.

Gershon, Michael D. *The Second Brain.* New York: HarperCollins, 1999.

Gomi, Taro. *Everyone Poops.* Brooklyn, New York: Kane/Miller Book Publishers, 1993.

Gottfried, Sara, MD. *The Hormone Cure: Reclaim Balance, Sleep and Sex Drive; Lose Weight; Feel Focused, Vital, and Energized Naturally.* New York: Scribner, 2013.

―――. *Younger: A Breakthrough Program to Reset Your Genes, Reverse Aging, and Turn Back the Clock Ten Years.* San Francisco: HarperOne, 2017.

Hedley, Gil, PhD. The Integral Anatomy Series. Integral Anatomy Productions, LLC, 2005.

Kern, Michael. *Wisdom in The Body.* London: Thorsons/HarperCollins, 2001.

van der Kolk, Bessel, MD. *The Body Keeps the Score: Brain, Mind, and Body in the Healing of Trauma.* New York: Penguin, 2015.

Knight, Rob and Buhler, Brendan. *Follow Your Gut, The Enormous Impact of Tiny Microbes.* New York: Simon & Schuster, 2015.

Kresser, Chris. *The Paleo Cure: Eat Right for Your Genes, Body Type, and Personal Health Needs.* New York/Boston/London: Little, Brown and Company, 2014.

Lau, D. C., trans. *Tao Te Ching.* New York: Penguin Books, 1963.

Lipski, Elizabeth. *Digestive Wellness.* Los Angeles: Keats Publishing, 1996.

Marin, Gilles. *Healing From Within with Chi Nei Tsang.* Berkeley, CA: North Atlantic Books, 1999.

Meyers, Amy. *The Autoimmune Solution: Prevent and Reverse the Full Spectrum of Inflammatory Symptoms and Diseases.* New York: HarperCollins, 2017.

Ostaseski, Frank. *The Five Invitations: Discovering What Death Can Teach Us About Living Fully.* New York: Flatiron Books, 2017.

Perlmutter, David, MD. *Brain Maker: The Power of Gut Microbes to Heal and Protect Your Brain–for Life.* New York/Boston/London: Little, Brown and Company, 2015.

Pitchford, Paul. *Healing with Whole Foods.* Berkeley, CA: North Atlantic Books, 1993.

Pollan, Michael. *The Omnivore's Dilemma: A Natural History of Four Meals.* New York: Penguin, 2007.

Porges, Stephen W. *The Polyvagal Theory: Neurophysiological Foundation of Emotions, Attachment, Communication, and Self-regulation.* New York: W. W. Norton & Company, 2011.

Romm, Aviva, MD. *The Adrenal Thyroid Revolution: A Proven 4-Week Program To Rescue Your Metabolism, Hormones, Mind, and Mood.* New York: HarperOne, 2017.

Roth, Geneen. *Women Food and God: An Unexpected Path to Almost Everything.* New York: Scribner, 2010.

Taubes, Gary. *The Case Against Sugar.* New York: Alfred A. Knopf, 2016.

Wentz, Izabella, Pharm.D, FASCP. *Hashimoto's Protocol: A 90-Day Plan for Reversing Thyroid Symptoms and Getting Your Life Back.* San Francisco: HarperCollins, 2017.

Yogi, Ramacharaka. *Science of Breath.* Chicago: Yogi Publication Society, 1905.

WEBSITES

http://americangut.org

https://avivaromm.com

https://chriskresser.com

https://draxe.com

http://gilhedley.com

https://www.nutrition.gov/shopping-cooking-meal-planning/food-labels

http://www.saragottfriedmd.com

For blood testing and health care support, see www.lifeextension.com

For comprehensive stool analysis, see www.doctorsdata.com

To contact the authors, please visit their website, www.allisonpost.com

INDEX

A

A&P study. *See* anatomy; physiology

Abdomen

  Belly Breathing and, 29

  combining abdominal massage with meditation, 5

  Connected Breathing and, 124–126

  exploring abdominal surface with Cat's Paw touch, 36–37

  lymph pumping, 38–40

  working on lower abdomen, 132–134

Abstraction, resulting from study, 158–159

Acid reflux, 97, 150

Action plan, for gut health

  blood tests and metabolic markers, 145–147

  comprehensive stool analysis, 149–151

  considerations of necessity of anatomy and physiology study, 157–160

  deepening embodiment practice, 156–157

  food elimination protocol, 151–154

  giving up sugars, 147–149

  making adjustments to plan, 154–156

  qualities needed to persist with, 144

  unhealthy patterns and, 141–143

Acupuncture, author studying holistic health regimes, 5

Adaptation

  making adjustments to action plan, 154–156

  qualities needed to persist with action plan, 144

Addiction

  complicated nature of, 106

  sugars and, 148–149

Adrenal glands, 113–114

Adrenaline, in fight or flight response, 113–114

Alcohol, moderation of use in medical response to adverse metabolic markers, 145–147

Allergies

  common food allergens, 152

  liver function and, 98

  microbiota imbalances and, 80

Allopathic medicine

  "fix it" approach in, 4

  intuition vs. medical research/science, 10

Anal sphincter, noticing tightness during breathing exercise, 92

Anatomy

  balancing mental knowledge with being grounded in body and feeling, 40

  study and, 157–160

Antacid overuse, 97

Antibiotics
 anecdote (Todd's story), 84
 overuse, 75
 as source of toxicity, 24
Anti-inflammatories, anecdote (Paul's story), 116
Arms, 51
Awareness. *See* self-awareness

B

Back
 anecdote (Paul's story), 116–118
 Belly Breathing and, 29
 Lateral Breathing and, 91
 low back pain, 115
 three-dimensional breathing, 110–111
 understanding the role of, 111–115
Bacteria
 ingesting microorganisms, 71
 as source of toxicity, 24
Balance, toward a balanced life, 141–144
Being, author's admonition to just be, 160
Belly area. *See* abdomen
Belly Breathing
 anecdote (Carol's story), 138
 anecdote (Joan's story), 41–42
 anecdote (Marguerite's story), 61–62
 anecdote (Todd's story), 86
 Connected Breathing and, 124
 exercise in, 29–31
 movement of diaphragm and, 32–33
 re-learning full, healthy breathing, 28
 what distinguishes Unwinding, 63
 why it is important, 27
Bellyaches
 digestive issues leading to more serious
  problems, 81–82
 impacting ability to focus, 142

Bile duct, understanding the digestive
 organs, 97
Birth control (IUD), infections related
 to, 2–3
Bladder
 organs of belly region, 13
 working on lower abdomen, 134
Blood
 circulatory system and, 79
 kidneys filtering, 111
 produced in bones, 135
 role of adrenals, 113–114
Blood pressure, 145
Blood tests
 adaptations in action plan and, 155
 value of, 145–147
Body. *See also* embodiment
 awareness during breathing exercise, 127
 being in tune with, 12
 brain chemistry reflecting state of, 18
 connective tissue as interlocking web, 35
 feeling bodily center, 92
 finding new ways to relate to, 4–7
 listening to, 64
 nourished by digestive process, 13
 potential for cellular and tissue
  regeneration, 143
 restoring holistic body-mind
  conversation, 21
 tissues, 14
Body language, 52–53
Bodywork, author studying holistic health
 regimes, 6
Bones
 awareness of, 134–135
 symptoms of release of tension,
  135–136
 touch techniques, 135
Book resource list, 161–163

Bowel movements and stools
    anecdote (Lisa's story), 102
    being conscious of what is taken in and
        what is eliminated, 60
    comprehensive stool analysis, 149–151
    constipation, diarrhea, irritable bowel
        syndrome, 59–60
    importance of observing stool, 57
    loose stools, 60
Brain chemistry, 17–18
Brain/nervous system
    circuit of healing, 38
    comprehensive stool analysis
        and, 150
    connection to muscles, 119–121
    gut and, 80–81
    integration and cooperation between
        three primary systems of body, 79
    restoring holistic body-mind
        conversation, 21
    self-help practice, 89
    three tubes (streaks) of embryo, 69–70
    unhealthy patterns and, 142–143
Breathing
    anecdote (Lisa's story), 104
    anecdote (Todd's story), 84
    belly. *See* Belly Breathing
    breathing, relaxing, and being happy, 1
    deepening embodiment practice, 156
    integrating the back, 110–111
    lateral. *See* Lateral Breathing
    leaning to limit, 128–129
    reverse breathing, 119
    three-dimensional. *See* Three-
        Dimensional Breathing
    understanding the role of the back,
        111–115
    unwinding via, 6
    what distinguishes Unwinding, 63

C

Carbohydrates, food elimination
    protocol, 152
Casein, common food allergens, 152
Cat's Paws touch
    anecdote (Todd's story), 85
    exercise connecting to large intestine,
        53–54
    exploring abdominal surface, 36–37
    lymph pumping, 39
    working on lower abdomen, 132–134
Cells, body potential for cellular
    regeneration, 143
Center, feeling bodily center, 92
Central nervous system, 70. *See also* brain/
    nervous system
Cesarean birth, imbalances due to, 75–76
Chemical sensitivity, 84
Chest area. *See also* ribs/rib cage
    anecdote (Carol's story), 138
    Connected Breathing and, 125–126
    reawakening and enlivening, 128
    skeletal connection of hips with, 135–136
    Three-Dimensional Breathing and, 110
Cholesterol, 145
Circuit of healing, 38
Circulatory system. *See* heart/circulatory
    system
Colon. *See* large intestine (colon)
Commitment, qualities needed to persist
    with action plan, 144
Common sense, in faulty perception of
    reality, 11
Compassion, 148
Connected Breathing
    bones and, 134–137
    as "do-it-yourself CPR," 129
    exercise, 124–127
    inner voice and, 128–130

Connected Breathing *(continued)*
  intercostals, 130–132
  lower abdomen, 132–134
  understanding, 127–128
Connective tissue, as interlocking web in
  body, 35
Constipation
  anecdote (Lisa's story), 102
  bowel movements and stools and,
  59–60
Contemplation, 157. *See also* meditation
Core fitness
  strengthening, 121
  Unwinding complements, 119
Co-relational care, 143
Cranial nerve pathways, between brain and
  gut-brain, 82
Craniosacral Therapy, 6

D

Dalkon Shield, infections related to birth
  control, 2–3
Deep sleep, 24, 142–143. *See also* sleep
Diaphragm
  expanded lateral breathing and, 92
  movement in breathing, 32–33
  psoas muscle connected to, 111
  restrictive behaviors creating patterns of
  tension, 129
  shape of relaxed, healthy diaphragm, 50
  understanding the colon, 55–56
Diarrhea, 59, 102
Diet
  anecdote (Lisa's story), 103–104
  anecdote (Marguerite's story), 61–62
  anecdote (Paul's story), 116
  food elimination protocol, 151–154
  giving up sugars, 147–149

importance of observing stool, 58–60
medical response to adverse metabolic
  markers, 145–147
search for proper diet, 14–15, 105–107
Digestion/digestive system
  anecdote (Marguerite's story), 61–62
  benefits of lateral breathing, 51
  body nourished by, 12–13
  digestion and assimilation of food, 150
  digestive issues leading to more serious
  problems, 82
  health emergency related to, 3
  illustration of digestive organs, 95–96
  importance of observing stool, 57
  microorganisms and, 77
  need for deeper understanding, 67–69
  organs of belly region and, 13
  process of, 70
  relaxation and, 15
  role of microorganisms in, 73–74
  stimulating the digestive organs, 92–94
  toxicity due to build-up of waste
  products, 14
  understanding the digestive organs, 95–99
  unhealthy patterns and, 142–143
  working on lower abdomen, 134
Discipline, in practice of Unwinding, 44–45
Disease
  importance of observing stool, 58
  preventative medicine, 51
Disembodiment
  being real in the present vs., 10
  study of emotional life and, 18
Doctors. *See also* allopathic medicine
  choosing, 150–151
  medical response to adverse metabolic
  markers, 145–147
Dopamine, 82
Drugs, as source of toxicity, 24

E

Eggs, common food allergens, 152

Elasticity, of muscles, 120

Electronic devices, over-stimulation and, 114–115

Elimination, 57. *See also* bowel movements and stools

Embodiment

deepening embodiment practice, 156–157

process of unwinding and settling, 7–8

self-help practice, 89

Unwinding as way to, 63–65

Embryo, three tubes (streaks) of, 69–72, 79

Emergence, finding new ways to relate to body, 4–7

Emergency, author's health crisis, 2–3

Emotions

addiction to sugar and, 148–149

anecdote (Carol's story), 138

bodily basis of, 19

as bodily functions not merely mind-based, 17–18

breaking cycles of psychological disharmony, 143

change occurs by working from emotional base not just mental, 20–21

conscious touch undoing emotional confusion, 133

inner voice expressing heart's desire, 128

integrating physical, emotional, and mental, 127

positive emotions, 20

reaction of colon to emotional stress, 56

Energy

author's health emergency, 3

digestion and, 12–13

liver function and, 98

Environment. *See* natural environment

Enzymes, digestive enzymes produced by pancreas, 98–99

Exercise

adaptations in action plan and, 156

lack of exercise as source of toxicity, 24

in medical response to adverse metabolic markers, 145–147

Exhalation

belly breathing, 30

Connected Breathing and, 124–125

with mouth closed, 63

movement of diaphragm and, 32–33

stimulating the digestive organs, 94

working on lower abdomen, 133

Expanded lateral breathing, 91–92

F

Fad diets, 105

Fallopian tubes, 134, 137–138

Farming, downside of modern practices, 74–75

Fascia

bodily basis of emotions, 19

navel as nexus of fascial system, 35

Fatigue, when to practice Unwinding, 44

Fats, food elimination protocol, 152

Fear, tension and, 134

Feel the wheel, 101

Fermented foods, as complement to probiotics, 155

Fiber

composition of foods, 152

elimination frequency and, 59

Fight or flight response, 113–114

Finger tips, circuit of healing, 38

Focused awareness, 156. *See also* self-awareness

Food
  adapting the action plan, 155
  anecdote (Lisa's story), 103–104
  assimilation, 78–79, 150
  benefits of whole, unprocessed foods, 101
  digestive process, 13
  downside of modern farming practices, 74
  energy from, 98
  food elimination protocol, 151–154
  food sensitivities and immune response, 80
  giving up sugars, 147–149
  GMOs (genetically modified organisms), 152–153
  importance of observing stool, 58–60
  microorganisms in digestive process, 77
  role of microorganisms in digestion, 73–74
  self-help practice, 89
Fungi
  ingesting microorganisms, 71
  testing for fungal infections, 150

G

Gallbladder
  benefits of lateral breathing, 51
  organs of belly region, 13
  stimulating the digestive organs, 92–94
  understanding the digestive organs, 97
Gastrointestinal system. See gut/gastrointestinal system
Glucose, blood tests and metabolic markers, 145
Gluten, common food allergens, 152
Glycogen, role of liver and, 98
GMOs (genetically modified organisms), in processed foods, 152–153
Grains, common food allergens, 152

Grief, bodily basis of emotions, 19
"gut matters," 67–69
Gut/gastrointestinal system
  antibiotics and, 75
  author's health emergency related to digestion, 3
  first line of defense against undesirable microorganisms, 73
  the gut brain, 78, 80–82
  gut/belly as home to emotions, 17
  imbalance of gut microbiota due to sugars, 99
  integrating back with belly, 111
  integration and cooperation between three primary systems of body, 79, 81–82
  letting it lead, 9
  plan for health of. See action plan, for gut health
  as root of health, 25
  specialized branch of nervous system, 80–81
  symptoms, problems, and diseases, 83
  three tubes (streaks) of embryo, 69–72
  viscera in, 13

H

Hands-on techniques, learning, 43
Happiness
  breathing, relaxing, and being happy, 1
  breathing and, 28
  health and healing and, 8, 12
Healing
  as dance not chore, 160
  happiness and, 8, 12
  massage and, 88
  medications work on symptoms not healing, 146
  working with loved ones, 45

Health
 being "real" in the present, 10
 giving up sugars, 147–149
 gut as root of, 25
 happiness and, 8, 12
 impact of microbiota and microbiome
  on, 142
 medications work on symptoms not
  healing, 146
 supermarkets and, 100–102
 unhealthy patterns and cycles associated
  with, 142–143
Heart emotions
 bodily basis of, 19
 inner voice expressing heart's desire, 128
Heart/circulatory system
 Connected Breathing and, 127
 immune response and, 80
 integration and cooperation between
  three primary systems of body, 79
 interconnectedness of heart with
  kidneys, 128
 three tubes (streaks) of embryo, 69–70
 unhealthy patterns and, 142–143
Height/weight ratio, 145
Helicobacter pylori, 60
Hemorrhoids, 103–104
Herbal medicine, 4
Hips
 Belly Breathing and, 29
 exploring abdominal surface with Cat's
  Paw touch, 36
 Lateral Breathing and, 91–92
 noticing tightness during breathing
  exercise, 91
 skeletal connection with chest, 135–136
 Three-Dimensional Breathing and, 110
 unwinding the navel, 34
 working on lower abdomen, 132–134

Holistic sensibility, 65
Hormones
 comprehensive stool analysis and, 150
 role of adrenals, 113–114

I

Ileocecal valve, 55
Imbalances, in microorganism culture
 cesarean birth and, 75–76
 comprehensive stool analysis checking
  for, 150
 digestive issues leading to more serious
  problems, 82
 due to sugars, 76, 99
 how to detect, 74–76
 origin of health issues, 155
 overview of, 72–74
 symptoms and impact on health, 80–81
Immune response
 circulatory system and, 79
 food sensitivities and, 80
Immunity/immune system, 95
 anecdote (Todd's story), 85
 comprehensive stool analysis and, 150
 declining diversity impacting, 74
 digestive issues leading to more serious
  problems, 82
 microorganisms and, 72–74
Infections
 antibiotics in treatment of, 2–3
 microorganisms and, 72–74
 testing for fungal infections, 150
Inflammation
 anti-inflammatories, 116
 markers for, 150
Inhalation
 belly breathing, 29–31
 Connected Breathing and, 124–125

Inhalation *(continued)*
  with mouth closed, 63
  movement of diaphragm and, 32–33
  stimulating the digestive organs, 94
  Three-Dimensional Breathing and, 109
  working on lower abdomen, 133
Inner voice
  feeling moved to sing and finding
    heartfelt happiness, 129–130
  reawakening and enlivening, 128
  restrictive behaviors and, 129
Inspire-ation, 128
Insulin, produced by pancreas, 99
Intercostals, Connected Breathing and,
  130–132
Internal organs. *See* vital organs
Intestine
  large. *See* large intestine (colon)
  small. *See* small intestine
Intuition
  allowing, 159
  following "gut instincts," 9–12
Irritable bowel syndrome, 59–60, 150
IUD (birth control), infections related to, 2–3

J
Jealousy, impact of emotions on gut, 17–18
Joint problems, 116
Just be, author's admonition, 160

K
Kefir, as complement to probiotics, 155
Kidneys
  interconnectedness with heart, 128
  organs of belly region, 13
  understanding the role of the back, 111

L
Lactose, common food allergens, 152

Large intestine (colon)
  connecting to, 53–54
  food assimilation, 79
  organs of belly region, 13
  shape of relaxed, healthy colon, 56
  understanding the colon, 55–57
Lateral Breathing
  Connected Breathing and, 124
  exercise, 48–49
  expanded lateral breathing, 91–92
  understanding, 50–53
Legs, noticing tightness during breathing
  exercise, 91
Life, toward a balanced life, 141–144
Listening
  to body, 64
  compassion and, 148
  important skill in choice of doctor,
    150–151
Liver
  benefits of lateral breathing, 51
  bodily basis of emotions, 19
  organs of belly region, 13
  stimulating the digestive organs,
    92–94
  understanding the digestive organs,
    97–98
Longevity, giving up sugars and, 148
Love, bodily basis of emotions, 19
Low back pain, 115
Lungs
  Belly Breathing and, 32
  Connected Breathing and, 124,
    127–128
  emotions and, 19
  panic/stress breathing and, 28, 33
Lymph, stimulating the digestive
  organs, 96
Lymph pumping, touch techniques,
  38–40

M

Macronutrients, 152

Martial arts, 119, 139–140

Massage. *See also* touch techniques

alternative to Unwinding, 88–89

author studying holistic health regimes, 4

combining with meditation, 5

intercostals, 130–132

Unwinding touch technique not a form of massage therapy, 63

working on lower abdomen, 132–134

Medical science. *See* allopathic medicine

Medications

anecdote (Lisa's story), 102

digestion and assimilation of, 81

in medical response to adverse metabolic markers, 146–147

supermarket products reflect health issues of many people, 100

symptom relief and, 149–150

Meditation

A&P study as an aid to, 159

combining abdominal massage with, 5

deepening embodiment practice, 156–157

Unwinding as complement to, 139–140

Unwinding as form of, 64, 89

Menstrual issues, 137–138

Mesentery

bodily basis of emotions, 19

organs of belly region, 13

Metabolic disorders/syndromes, 145–147

Metabolic markers, 145–147

Metabolism

author's health emergency, 3

benefits of lateral breathing, 51

role of adrenals, 113–114

Microbiome, 78, 142

Microbiota. *See* microorganisms

Microorganisms

allergies and food sensitivities, 80

comprehensive stool analysis checking for imbalances in, 150

gut-brain and, 81–82

health and, 76–77

how to detect imbalances, 74–76

imbalances in microbiota as origin of health issues, 155

impact on health, 142

infection, immunity, and imbalance, 72–74

ingesting, 71

microbiome, 78

sugars and, 149

Milk, common food allergens, 152

Mind. *See also* brain/nervous system

integrating physical, emotional, and mental, 127

study of emotional life and, 18

Modern medicine. *See* allopathic medicine

Movement

enhanced lateral movement, 52–53

freeing up, 111–112

muscle tonicity and, 119

pleasurable, 23

springs from center not just physical, 21–23

Muscles

connection to nervous system, 119–121

elasticity of, 120

pain generally registered in muscles and tendons, 136

psoas muscles, 111, 133

tonicity, 119

N

Natural environment

decline of diversity in, 74

disassociation from, 75

Navel
anecdote (Carol's story), 138
anecdote (Joan's story), 40–42
expanded lateral breathing and, 91–92
reasons for working on, 35
Unwinding exercise, 34–36
Nervous system. *See* brain/nervous system
Neurotransmitters, 82

O
Oils, common food allergens, 152
Organs. *See* vital organs
Overwork
qualities of modern life, 114–115
as source of toxicity, 24
when to practice Unwinding, 44

P
Pain
anecdote (Carol's story), 137
anecdote (Paul's story), 116–118
generally registered in muscles and
tendons, 136
low back pain, 115
temporary relief vs. real change,
141–142
Pancreas
benefits of lateral breathing, 51
measuring pancreatic juices, 150
organs of belly region, 13
understanding the digestive organs,
98–99
Parasites
comprehensive stool analysis checking
for, 150
as source of toxicity, 24
Patience, qualities needed to persist with
action plan, 144

Peanuts, common food allergens, 152
Pelvic girdles. *See* chest area; hips
Pelvic inflammatory disease, 3
Pelvis
connecting to large intestine, 54
expanded lateral breathing and, 91–92
Three-Dimensional Breathing and,
110–111
working with intercostals, 132
working with lower abdomen, 133
Peritoneum, 13
Physical, integrating with emotional and
mental, 127. *See also* body
Physiology
balancing mental knowledge with being
grounded in body and feeling, 40
considerations of necessity of anatomy
and physiology study, 157–160
cycles of physiological disharmony can
be broken/changed, 143
Pollution, toxicity due to, 24
Present, being "real" in the present, 10
Preventative medicine, 51
Probiotics, 155
Proteins, food elimination protocol, 152
Psoas muscles
movement and, 111
working on lower abdomen, 133

Q
Qigong
antidotes to beliefs and over-
mentalizing, 160
reverse breathing, 119
Unwinding as complement to, 139–140

R
Rectum, 55

Relaxation
   breathing, relaxing, and being happy, 1
   deepening embodiment practice, 156
   digestion and, 15
   key in food taking, 155
   muscles and, 119
   over-stimulation as quality of modern
      life, 114–115
   self-help practice, 89
   via breath, 6
Remedies, supermarket products reflecting
   common health issues, 100
Reproductive organs
   anecdote (Carol's story), 137–138
   organs of belly region, 13
   working on lower abdomen, 134
Resources
   books, 161–163
   websites, 163
Respiratory problems, 98
Rest, 156
Ribs/rib cage. *See also* chest area
   anecdote (Carol's story), 138
   Connected Breathing and, 124, 126
   exercise connecting to large intestine,
      53–54
   expanded lateral breathing and, 92
   exploring abdominal surface with Cat's
      Paw touch, 36
   Lateral Breathing and, 48–49, 92
   massaging intercostal area, 130–132
   stimulating the digestive organs, 93–94
   symptoms of restriction, 51–52
   understanding lateral breathing, 50

S

Science, as tool not replacement or
   alternative to personal intuition, 10, 12
Second Brain, 81

Self-awareness
   anecdote (Lisa's story), 104–105
   being aware of body during breathing
      exercise, 127
   of bones, 134–135
   deepening embodiment practice, 156
   development of, 88–89
   feeling the back, 109
   of spine, 135
Self-help practice
   anecdote (Lisa's story), 104–105
   development of, 88–89
Serotonin, 82
Shellfish, common food allergens, 152
Shiatsu, 5
Side bends, in stretching routines, 52
Skin
   circuit of healing, 38
   reasons for working on skin, 37–38
Sleep
   lack of deep sleep as source of
      toxicity, 24
   regeneration during, 120
   stress and, 142–143
Slow down, 156
Small intestine
   food assimilation, 79
   organs of belly region, 13
   toxicity and, 14
   working on lower abdomen, 134
Spine
   awareness of in Connected Breathing,
      135
   loosening process and, 137
Spleen
   benefits of lateral breathing, 51
   organs of belly region, 13
   understanding the digestive organs,
      96–97

Stimulation, over-stimulation as quality of
modern life, 114–115
Stomach
author's health emergency, 3
benefits of lateral breathing, 51
common nature of stomach problems, 4
organs of belly region, 13
Stomach acids, 150
Stools. *See* bowel movements and stools
Stress/tension
anecdote (Carol's story), 129
fear and, 134
fight or flight response, 113–114
importance of observing stool, 57
muscle in constant state of contraction,
120
navigating, 1
numerous vectors in contemporary
world, 68
reaction of colon to, 56
self-help practice, 89
sleep and, 142–143
sources of, 23–25
symptoms of release by bones, 135–136
toxicity from tension, 14
unraveling sources of, 7
Stretching routines, 52
Study, of anatomy and physiology, 157–160
Sugars
giving up, 147–149
microbiota imbalances and, 76, 99
Supermarkets
anecdote (Lisa's story), 103
health and, 100–102
Supplements
anecdote (Lisa's story), 102–103
cautions in use of, 155
downside of reliance on, 101
Surgery, as source of toxicity, 24

Symptoms
medications suppressing, 100–101
medications work on symptoms not
healing, 146

T

T'ai chi
reverse breathing, 119
Unwinding as complement to, 139–140
Taoism, 5
Tendons, pain registered in, 136
Tension. *See* stress/tension
Thorax. *See* chest area
Three-Dimensional Breathing
Connected Breathing and, 124
integrating the back, 110–111
overview of, 109–110
understanding the role of the back,
111–115
Throat, 128
Tissues
of the body, 14
body potential for cellular and tissue
regeneration, 143
examples of bodily basis of emotions, 19
Tonicity, muscle strength and, 119
Touch techniques. *See also* Cat's Paws touch
anecdote (Carol's story), 138
anecdote (Paul's story), 117–118
anecdote (Todd's story), 85
effectiveness of delicate touch, 38
exploring abdominal surface with Cat's
Paw touch, 36–37
increasing blood flow to low back and
adrenals, 115
intercostals, 130–132
lymph pumping, 38–40
reasons for working on skin, 37–38
stimulating the digestive organs, 92–94

Unwinding the navel, 34–36
what distinguishes Unwinding, 63
working on lower abdomen, 132–134
working with bones, 135
Toxicity
belly breathing removing, 31
pollution causing, 24
from tension, 14
Traditional Chinese Medicine, 5
Triglycerides, 145
Trunk, benefits of loosening sides of, 51–52

U

Unwinding
abs and core focus versus, 118–120
anecdote (Carol's story), 137–138
anecdote (Joan's story), 40–42
anecdote (Lisa's story), 102–105
anecdote (Marguerite's story), 61–62
anecdote (Paul's story), 116–118
anecdote (Todd's story), 85–87
Belly Breathing exercise, 29–31
comparing with other systems, 62–65
Connected Breathing exercise, 124–128
in dealing with stress, 25
dealing with trauma, 6
effectiveness of delicate touch, 38
as embodiment process, 7–8
exercise connecting to large intestine,
53–54
expanded lateral breathing, 91–92
exploring abdominal surface with Cat's
Paw touch, 36–37
intermediate steps, 47
Lateral Breathing exercise, 48–49
lymph pumping, 38–40
massage not alternative to, 88–89
the navel, 34–36

reasons for working on skin, 37–38
re-learning full, healthy breathing,
27–28
restoring holistic body-mind
conversation, 21
self-help practice, 89
stimulating the digestive organs, 92–94
understanding lateral breathing, 50–53
understanding the colon, 55–57
understanding the digestive organs,
95–99
when and how much to practice, 43–45
yoga complementing, 139–140
Ureters, 13
Urinary systems, 70

V

Vagus nerve, 82
Viruses
ingesting microorganisms, 71
as source of toxicity, 24
Viscera
being in touch with, 15–16
bodily basis of emotions, 19
circuit of healing, 38
Connected Breathing and, 127–128
organs of belly region, 13
understanding the role of the back,
111–112
Visceral Manipulation, 5
Vital organs
of belly region, 13
benefits of lateral breathing, 51
Connected Breathing and, 127–128
stimulating the digestive organs, 92–94
understanding the digestive organs,
95–99
Vitamins, 77

W

Waist-to-hip circumference ratio, 145
Water
  elimination frequency and, 59
  value as main beverage, 105
Website resources, 163
Weight
  maintaining healthy weight, 153
  microbiota imbalances and, 80
Weight loss diets, 105
Wheat, common food allergens, 152
Worry, impact of emotions on gut, 17

Y

Yeast, testing for imbalances in, 150
Yoga
  anecdote (Paul's story), 116
  as antidote to beliefs and over-
    mentalizing, 160
  author studying holistic health
    regimes, 6
  Unwinding as complement to, 139–140
Yogurt, as complement to probiotics, 155

ABOUT THE AUTHORS

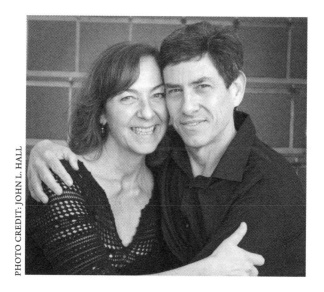

PHOTO CREDIT: JOHN L. HALL

ALLISON POST is a somatic educator and integrative medicine health coach with more than thirty years of experience helping individuals rediscover inherent health and happiness. Her specialty is to draw upon the deep wells of both modern and traditional medical wisdom to help people incorporate breath, gastrointestinal balance, embodiment skills, and movement into their daily lives with presence and joy.

STEPHEN CAVALIERE is a writer with an interest in the history and practice of physical culture. He has completed courses with Outward Bound and the National Outdoor Leadership School, and enjoys trekking in Europe and Asia, studying languages, and learning how others approach exercise and fitness.

The authors are currently creating online course offerings and writing a book about love.

About North Atlantic Books

North Atlantic Books (NAB) is an independent, nonprofit publisher committed to a bold exploration of the relationships between mind, body, spirit, and nature. Founded in 1974, NAB aims to nurture a holistic view of the arts, sciences, humanities, and healing. To make a donation or to learn more about our books, authors, events, and newsletter, please visit www.northatlanticbooks.com.

North Atlantic Books is the publishing arm of the Society for the Study of Native Arts and Sciences, a 501(c)(3) nonprofit educational organization that promotes cross-cultural perspectives linking scientific, social, and artistic fields. To learn how you can support us, please visit our website.